PLAGUES AND PANDEMICS

Wuhan. Covid-19. So what's new? This virus maybe, but not epidemics and pandemics.

They ended many prehistoric civilisations suddenly, leaving entire cities undamaged to mystify archeologists. Plague in Athens killed 30% of the population in 430–26 BCE. In 541 CE plague claimed several thousand lives a day inside the walls of Constantinople.

It returned to kill 50 million people in Europe in 1346–53, visiting London forty times in the following 300 years, of which the outbreak 1665–66 was known as the Great Plague. Closer to our times, when it returned to China in 1894 it claimed between twelve and fifteen million lives in Asia, before finally dying down in the 1950s after visiting San Francisco and New York. It also hit Madagascar in 2014, and the Congo and Peru. Infected fleas from rats on merchant ships were originally blamed for spreading it, but modern scientists have a more worrying explanation why the plague spread so fast.

There have been many other killer pandemics. The misnamed Spanish 'flu of 1918–20 killed up to 100 million people. The new coronavirus Covid-19 is NOT the most lethal pandemic so far.

Chillingly, historian Douglas Boyd lists many other sub-microscopic killers still waiting for the resurgence of tourism and trade to bring them right into our lives.

PLAGUES AND PANDEMICS

Black Death, Coronaviruses and Other Killer Diseases Throughout History

Douglas Boyd

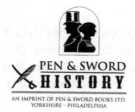

PEN & SWORD **HISTORY**

AN IMPRINT OF PEN & SWORD BOOKS LTD.
YORKSHIRE – PHILADELPHIA

First published in Great Britain in 2021 by
PEN AND SWORD HISTORY
An imprint of
Pen & Sword Books Ltd
Yorkshire – Philadelphia

Copyright © Douglas Boyd, 2021

ISBN 978 1 39900 518 0

Typeset in Times New Roman 11.5/14 by
SJmagic DESIGN SERVICES, India.
Printed and bound in the UK by CPI Group (UK) Ltd.

Pen & Sword Books Limited incorporates the imprints of Atlas, Archaeology,
Aviation, Discovery, Family History, Fiction, History, Maritime, Military, Military
Classics, Politics, Select, Transport, True Crime, Air World, Frontline Publishing,
Leo Cooper, Remember When, Seaforth Publishing, The Praetorian Press,
Wharncliffe Local History, Wharncliffe Transport, Wharncliffe True Crime and
White Owl.

For a complete list of Pen & Sword titles please contact
PEN & SWORD BOOKS LIMITED
47 Church Street, Barnsley, South Yorkshire, S70 2AS, England
E-mail: enquiries@pen-and-sword.co.uk
Website: www.pen-and-sword.co.uk

Or
PEN AND SWORD BOOKS
1950 Lawrence Rd, Havertown, PA 19083, USA
E-mail: Uspen-and-sword@casematepublishers.com
Website: www.penandswordbooks.com

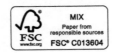

Contents

Glossary

antibiotic – in medicine, a substance produced from micro-organisms which has the ability to inhibit the growth of, or destroy, micro-organisms producing disease

antibody – a defensive substance produced in the body to combat infection, intrusion of a foreign body, substance or parasite

arbovirus – acronym of ARhropod-BOrne VIRUS

arthropod – a flea, tick, spider, millipede, centipede or other species which may bite or inject infected blood-thinners into a mammalian victim

bacillus – another name for any disease-causing bacterium

bacterium – a class of micro-organism, larger than viruses, and therefore identified with early microscopes

BP – of dates, Before the Present

BCE – of dates, Before the Common Era – formerly BC for *before Christ* was used

CE – of dates, in the Common Era – formerly AD for *anno domini* was used

Enzootic – of a disease, surviving in another animal species

filovirus – a threadlike virus of the group that includes Ebola and Marburg fevers

host – an animal or other species that supports a dangerous bacterium or virus which may attack humans

immune system – humans possess three major types of immunity: the humoral uses antibodies already in circulation to attack and remove pathogens in the bloodstream; the mucosal protects from pathogens in the small intestine and the lungs; and the cellular, which detects infected cells and destroys them.

MRSA - methicillin-resistant staphylococcus aurea, a bacterium that has acquired resistance to many over-prescribed antibiotic medicines

Parish – the area served by a church, which in medieval London also served as an administrative district

pathogen – an organism or substance that causes disease

petechia – a small red or purple spot in the skin caused by a ruptured blood vessel

plasmodia – single-celled protozoa that cause malaria and other diseases in animals and birds; four species multiply in human blood after the bite of an infected mosquito – *malariae, falciparum, vivax* and *ovale.* retrovirus – a virus that has RNA as its genetic material, and uses an enzyme called reverse transcriptase to become part of the host cells and replicate there

rickettsia – a micro-organism found in lice and ticks which, when transferred to humans, causes typhus

vector – the means or route by which a pathogen enters the victim's body

WHO – World Health Organisation

zoonotic – of disease, caught from another animal species

Introduction

There is nothing new about epidemic diseases. The Greek word *epidemia* is derived from *epi* meaning 'on' and *demos* meaning the whole people or country, and it pre-dates Hippocrates, who used it more than 2,000 years ago. A *pandemia* was a disease that spread all over a region or, by extension, the whole known world. However, most people suppress unpleasant memories, which is why the Covid-19 coronavirus pandemic caused such a shock in early 2020. People who play word games and are given 'pandemic' immediately see 'panic' in it, and many of the world's governments certainly panicked when Covid-19 arrived.

Yet, during the lifetime of many readers of this book a variant killer 'flu virus designated H3N2 was first recorded in the British colony of Hong Kong in July 1968 – leading to its common name of Hong Kong 'flu. The Chinese Communist government of the time suppressing news of any negative event, its probable origin on the mainland is undocumented in any way that foreigners have been able to access. Going pandemic, H3N2 certainly killed a million people worldwide and is thought to have caused up to three times as many additional deaths in Third World countries where medicine was less developed, mortality from all causes more frequent and records ill-kept. The disease was allowed to spread, few preventive measures being taken until a vaccine became available after four months. But the H3N2 virus continued causing more deaths in 1969–70, and still resurfaces with many variants in each 'flu season.

The so-called Asian 'flu due to virus H2N2 almost certainly started in China a decade earlier. Because of government censorship on the Chinese mainland, the first reports came out of Singapore during February 1957. This virus certainly killed a recorded 1.1 million people, although the World Health Organisation estimated total deaths to be nearer 2 million. We talk glibly about viruses today, but the word *virus* is Latin, meaning a poison like snake venom, and people tend to fear all viruses. Some are so small they cannot be seen by optical microscopes and a few are larger than the smallest bacteria; some attack bacteria, which is surely a good thing for us. And two viruses named syncytin-1 and syncytin-2 are believed to have stopped our *very* remote female ancestors' immune systems from attacking foetuses as foreign bodies – bestowing on those ancestors the extraordinary advantage of being able to transport the unborn offspring inside their bodies, instead of leaving them somewhere in a nest as birds and reptiles have to do. A fascinating article by David Quammen is downloadable from https://www.nationalgeographic.com/magazine/2021/02/viruses-can-cause-great-harm-but-we-could-not-live-without-them-feature / from the February 2021 *National Geographic* magazine all about these minute but powerful protein-coated particles of DNA or RNA.

Yet, how many of us – apart from medical professionals – can clearly recall even 'flu epidemics of a few years ago? Most European readers will have heard of the Black Death plague in the fourteenth and seventeenth centuries that killed off between a third and a half of the population of Europe and many millions elsewhere. So horrific were its physical manifestations and so disruptive was it of normal life that it is probably the best-remembered pandemic. How many know that this was not the first pandemic? And what about the third bubonic plague, much nearer our own time, which began in China in 1855 and killed about 12.5 million, mostly in Asia? At least 10 million died in India alone, where British attempts to impose Western medical practice and vaccination were resisted for religious and other reasons by the native population.

Alarmingly, the WHO states that this pandemic continued as late as 1960, after when a much decreased number of deaths continued to occur. And they still do, but only in the Third World. However, a Reuters report of 14 November 2002 recorded the case of Lucinda Marker and her partner, the lawyer John Tull, who were hospitalised with bubonic plague in New York. With the help of antibiotics, she recovered and left hospital after a few days, but he was more seriously ill, probably because he was diabetic. When his kidneys began to fail, Tull was put into an induced coma, during which Ms Marker authorised surgeons to amputate his legs below the knee, to prevent the infection spreading. He spent a total of 224 days in hospital before being pronounced fit to leave, fitted with prosthetic lower legs.

This was shortly after anthrax spores had been mailed to prominent Americans following the 9/11 attacks, so many people believed that Tull and his partner were victims of bioterrorism until it was revealed that they had come to New York from their home in New Mexico, where they had caught the disease from fleas migrating to human hosts from dead rodents on their property, probably prairie dogs. About a dozen cases of this plague are diagnosed in humans from the rural states of southwestern USA each year, although mostly in a 'plague season' between May and September, and particularly in the region known as the Four Corners, where four state boundaries meet – they are, clockwise from the northwest corner to the southwest, Utah, Colorado, New Mexico and Arizona. This area is also a reservoir of another plague very dangerous for humans, of which more later.

Other rodents that carry the plague pathogen are turbots, marmots, squirrels, gerbils and roughly 200 other mammalian species including camels – and chickens. The rodents' fleas also migrate to domestic animals, especially dogs and cats, which sniff around the burrows and then return to the family home, acting as plague-carriers unknown to their owners. The pathogen now designated *Y. pestis* is today widely distributed among wild rodent populations in Eastern Europe, Asia, Africa and the Americas. In inhabited areas, plague-carrying rats feed on refuse and garbage, so inadequate cleaning of street markets makes a rich source of food for them. They also find rich pickings in the fodder of farm animals, so that farmers and farm labourers are at higher risk than others.

Also resident in the Four Corners area of the United States lives the pretty white-footed deermouse. Unimpressed by its delicate appearance, the Navajo people, who lived here before white Americans took away their land, kept well away from rodents, including this one. They knew something that modern science has only recently discovered: that this species is host to a number of hantaviruses which can be fatal to humans.

Chapter 1

Ancient Plagues

Today, improved personal hygiene reduces the risk of contamination, but in the past people washed rarely and often slept in their day-clothes, providing a secure home for their fleas, especially *pulex irritans*, which prefers human and swine blood.

There are uncountable trillions of bacteria living on the planet, many of them inside us in a symbiotic relationship where they cause no harm. But many dangerous bacteria and viruses pre-existed mankind, with evidence of their presence found in fossils of dinosaurs and other creatures that lived millions of years before the evolution of our species. The skeleton of a Jurassic crocodile from 14 million years ago showed infection in the pelvis, with metastases in the femur, the sacral vertebrae and the palate. Many fossils show bone necrosis and subsequent hyperstoses (excessive bone growth, a marker of past infections); evidence of bacterial infection is widespread. When our remote primate ancestors arrived on the scene, they were afflicted by mites, fleas, ticks, flies and worms and were parisited by protozoa, fungi and bacteria plus several hundred arboviruses able to jump species with often fatal results. These included yellow fever, dengue and chikungunya, vectored by tick or mosquito bites.[1] Variants of these still lie in wait as mankind continues to intrude into, and destroy, the warm and humid rain forests.[2]

This is where it gets difficult. Most people have heard of the Black Death as a medieval plague. Wrong. An extraordinary multi-university research programme headed by Aida Andrades Valtueña from the Archeogenetic Department of the Max Planck Institute in Jena, Germany, literally dug up evidence that bubonic plague visited Europe at least as early as 5,000 years ago. In 2018, evidence of the plague bacillus was uncovered in a prehistoric tomb in Sweden also dated to 3,000 BCE – the Late Neolithic and Early Bronze Age. Quite conceivably, it arrived in Europe even earlier, but if so evidence is lacking, so far. Meticulous archeobiological research was based on

1

DNA analysis of teeth removed from skeletons from this period, in or on which they found traces of the plague bacillus, now known as *Yersinia pestis* or *Y. pestis* in short.[3]

In Russia, remains of humans killed by *Y. pestis* dug up from the grasslands of the steppes bears out coincidences with Russian linguistics. For example, the word for 'to find' is *nakhodit'*, which means literally to walk onto something before you can see it, the implication being that the originators of the language lived in the long grasses of the steppes, where a lost object would be difficult to see even a few paces away.

Here we have to stop. There was not one plague bacillus, but various species in the genus *Y. pestis*. It is a multi-host and multi-vector pathogen involving more than 200 species of wild rodents as hosts and over eighty species of fleas as vectors. The full genome of *Y. pestis* is about 5.6 million base pairs long. A base pair is the fundamental unit of double-stranded nucleic acids, so that is quite a lot. The fragments that researchers have had to deal with from archeological discovery are rarely even fifty to seventy-five base pairs long and may be contaminated in the ground, during collection or in the laboratory. This makes it quite understandable that the research of the late 1990s and early 2000s provided few final answers. However, in 2004 another diagnostic process using a protein assay that tested for an antigen produced uniquely by *Y. pestis* proved useful in determining its presence, not only in modern samples and epidemiological surveys, but also in historical samples.

In 2015, more advanced research seemed to indicate that the bacterium in question was not capable of causing plague in the Bronze Age, and had evolved from *Y. pseudotuberculosis* between 2,600 and 28,000 years BP (before the present).[4] The relevant Report by M. Rasmussen et al (2010) suggested that *Y. pestis* did not fully adapt as a flea-borne mammalian pathogen until the beginning of the first millennium BCE – and precipitated the historically recorded plagues. The present author can hardly argue with the Rasmussen report, compiled by thirty-one highly qualified scientists, but ...

Meanwhile, studies reporting success by the former methods kept appearing until it was announced that the complete genome of *Y. pestis* had been assembled from fourteenth-century samples. Plague was an important factor in the medieval history of Western Europe. It also affected the Middle East, Russia, India, North, East and Central Africa, where it still remains in enzootic foci, primarily in rodents. They don't have to be rats. In the US even cute little marmots and prairie dogs can be plague vectors, as can seventy-five other mammalian species.

Reading the literature, it seems at first that there are four forms of plague, but the names refer to the manner in which the pathogen enters a victim's body. Bubonic plague enters through the bite of a flea or other insect, itself infected by the infected blood of a rodent or other mammalan species it has parasited, or by abrasion or a cut in the skin. It swiftly reaches the lymphatic system, causing among other effects the dark swellings, or buboes, over the affected glands. The disease is called pneumonic plague when infection occurs through inhalation of droplets from the cough or sneeze of an infected person or animal – even domestic cats and dogs. The pathogen in this case primarily targets the victim's lungs and respiratory system. When the pathogen first invades the vessels and organs involved in the circulation of blood, by entering through a cut or wound, it produces septicaemic plague, which kills fast. The term gastrointestinal plague is used when infection is via infected food or drink. Whatever the name, the disease is essentially the same, but manifests its presence differently.

The plague pathogen is known scientifically as *Yersinia pestis*, an offshoot thousands of years ago from the *pseudotuberculosis* bacillus. One of the alarming facts about viruses and bacteria that cause infection in humans is that they evolve rapidly in human terms because the life cycle of a microorganism is so short. So a bacterium can swiftly become resistant to antibiotics that formerly cured it. A classic example is the hospital infection MRSA, standing for methicillin-resistant staphylococcus aurea, which just shrugs off treatment by antibiotics. And, as we found out in 2020 the Covid-19 virus has produced many variants.

In 1898 plague returned to the Indian sub-continent and, in repeated outbreaks, carried off 12.5 million people in the following decade.[5] A century later the official report to the Indian government on the 1994 plague in Beed and Surat traces plague in India back to roughly 1500 BCE, as mentioned in the Hindu history Bhagavata Purana, originally written in about 3100 BCE and revised many times since. The 1994 outbreak seemed to be a consequence of a violent earthquake in the previous year that caused millions of rats to re-locate – and die. So many, in fact that it seemed they had rained down from the sky. Their fleas transferred to human hosts, whose blood was tested for antibodies in Delhi. *Only* 460 people died, however. Did the others have some immunity? Swiftly afterwards, monsoon rains caused flooding in Surat, north of Mumbai, where people suffering pneumonic plague overloaded the hospitals with symptoms of high fever, respiratory problems and coughing up blood.

The instant that the word *plague* was uttered in loudspeaker announcements, people, both sick and healthy, started to leave the city, heading for the homes of relatives hundreds of miles away. Among those departing were many doctors. International airlines shut down their flights from India, but not until many travellers had been tested at their destinations for symptoms of fever. In New York, four were diagnosed with malaria and one with typhoid fever, examples of the dangers of international air travel. Trading partners of the sub-continent refused to buy Indian foodstuffs. The Indian government sprayed hundreds of tons of DDT and other insecticides around the infected area and hundreds of thousands of tetracycline tablets were handed out to the people reporting sick.

Biologist Christopher Wills travelled to India soon afterwards and was told that the drugs and spraying had apparently contained the outbreak, with opinions divided among health care professionals as to whether this had been plague, or not. Two letters to *The Lancet* from the All-India Institute of Medical Sciences in New Delhi, questioned the plague theory. Wills visited the All-India Medical College at Vellore in the southern Indian state of Tamil Nadu, where microbiologist T. Jacob John did likewise, pointing out that the disease in Beed could have been tularaemia, which can mimic the swollen lymph nodes without having the mortality of plague. Dr John also considered that the disease in Surat might have been due to *pseudomonas pseudomallei* which causes meliodosis and can produce symptoms like those of pneumonic plague. But when he and his colleagues wished to present their arguments to the Indian Association of Microbiologists in Poona, he was refused permission by the Minister for Health of Maharashtra state, which includes Beed. A furious altercation ensued, after which a reluctant permission was given for the team from Vellore to make its presentation.[6]

An even more confusing explanation of the doubt about the 1994 plague – if it was plague – was given to Wills in Delhi by K.B. Sharma, a regional advisor for the WHO. According to him, the first attempts to isolate and identify the bacillus that had caused the disease failed due to laboratory technicians incubating the specimens for insufficient time for them to develop! Dr R.C. Panda had worked round the clock for three weeks caring for the victims of this outbreak and found streptomycin and tetracycline effective in curing the sufferers with high fever and acute chest pain who were coughing up blood from their lungs. He was convinced they were suffering from pneumonic plague, but complained that the WHO had never sought his opinion. Every Indian specialist and official whom Wills consulted seemed to disagree with the others.[7]

If diagnosing modern outbreaks of plague and plague-like diseases can be so confusing, what about diagnosing ancient plagues? In the late twentieth century, work by German scientists analysing skeletal DNA of two sixth-century plague victims in Alterneding, Bavaria, enabled them to confirm the presence of *Y. pestis* in a tooth of a young female victim, as reported in the professional journal *Molecular Biology and Evolution*. American researchers led by microbial geneticist Dave Wagner from Northern Arizona University, working on another plague skeleton dug up nearby, afterwards reconstructed the genome of the pathogen and found it was different from the strain that caused the Justinian plague, identifying thirty new mutations and structural rearrangements.[8] So it seems that the cause designated *Y. pestis* is more versatile than formerly believed. What the implications are, we may yet find out.

Whole genome research suggests that all variants of the bacterium have evolved from an ancient common ancestor. Only three of these are able to infect humans: *Y. pestis, Y. pseudotuberculosis* and *Y. enterocolitica*. The last-named reaches the victim by the consumption of infected food or water and usually induces severe gastroenteritis. *Y. pestis* however is vectored (i.e. brought to the human victim) by an arthropod such as the flea or by cough droplets, depending on its form. It has three forms. The bubonic form is the commonest and generally transmitted to a human host by the bites of an infected flea when that flea injects some anticoagulant saliva to enable human blood to be sucked up through its narrow stylets. In the saliva is some of the proliferating bacterium blocking the throat of the flea, which it is desperate to get rid of.

Where did the flea get infected? That is something which people virtually devoid of science, and lacking any magnification to examine these tiny insects of 1.5 to 3.2 mm long, worked out by common sense centuries ago. The flea becomes infected by sucking blood from an infected rodent. Once in the human victim's bloodstream, the regurgitated pathogen reproduces at an alarming rate producing in a few days the typical pus-filled buboes – dark swellings on the skin over the lymphatic glands – and by invading organs such as the liver and spleen.[9]

The septicaemic form of *Y. pestis* is also contracted by the bite of an infected flea. Symptoms include fever, chills, abdominal pain, diarrhoea and vomiting, bleeding from the mouth and blackening of body tissues. Medically uncontrollable haemorrhaging often causes death within twenty-four hours of the flea-bite. The pneumonic form of the plague needs no flea as vector, and infects its victims through sputum droplets in the air coughed or sneezed up by an infected person. Again, people worked this out for themselves centuries ago. In this case, the pathogen fills the lungs of the human victim with fluid, eventually preventing breathing. It too can kill within twenty-four hours of the flea-bite.[10]

It has been pointed out that early documentation of plague by Boccaccio, Procopius and Samuel Pepys, to mention but three, does not mention rats and fleas, but this may be because rats and fleas were so ubiquitous in those times that people took no special notice of them.

Since intra-special contact is required for an epidemic, we cannot know how much these pathogens bothered ancient humans in the Stone Age and Early Bronze Age hunter-gatherer stage of our evolution. At the end of the last Ice Age, when the enormously heavy mile-thick ice sheet that covered the British Isles melted, allowing the land to spring up in places by several feet, there was no vegetation in the ice-eroded landscape. Once that took root with wind-blown seeds from the European continent and seeds that had survived under the ice, many species of herbivores crossed the land-bridge that became the North Sea 12,000 years ago.

Predator species followed the herbivores. In the Neolithic, or Late Stone age, these predators included small groups of hunter-gatherer humans until there were an estimated 2,000 individuals roaming the more hospitable regions of what is now England and Wales. Each group had only intermittent contact with others because a different group might kill all the males and take the females prisoner. Cannibalism of human captives was also commonly practised at this stage. We do not know how many people died from infection during this phase of evolution, but the conditions were not favourable to epidemics. Yet the plague bacilli did not die off; they seem to have a frightening tendency to, as it were, hibernate and emerge when conditions are favourable for them.

An odd reference to a plague afflicting the Hebrews in their forty-year wanderings after escaping from Egypt can be found in the Old Testament. The Bible, is, of course, not history. So dating a Biblical event or person requires cross-referencing. Moses is reputed to have lived c. 1300 BCE and a contemporary of his named Pinchas or Phineas is credited with stopping a plague about that date, during the forty years' wandering in the wilderness that Moses decreed so that all adults who had grown up in Egyptian slavery would die off before he settled the Hebrews as free people in Canaan – the land of milk and honey that would have to be won by warfare against the Canaanites.

As customary with primitive people, the Hebrews considered the plague that afflicted them, killing 24,000 to be a punishment sent by their God, in this case for their menfolk having sexual relations with Midianite women while their wanderings took them into the land of Moab and Shittim, east of the Jordan river.[11] Pinchas, son of Eleazar the son of Aaron, made his point by driving a spear into the chest of the offending Hebrew Zimri who was sinning with the Midianite woman Cozbi, whom Pinchas stabbed in the belly. The Midianites were a related Semitic people, so it is unclear why their women were off-limits. Indeed, one of Moses' own wives was a Midianite named Tsiporah. It sounds like a case of 'Don't do what I do. Do what I tell you.'

The problem for historians is that the story of Pinchas was orally transmitted for several centuries before being written down, the Hebrew alphabet only being created c. 800 BCE. So we have no information about the specific nature of this plague. At the time, there were said to be 601,730 Hebrews in all the tribes, so losing 24,000 was not critical. To find food supplies for more than half a million nomads and their grazing animals including sheep, goats and cattle, seems impossible, and would account for any 'invaded' peoples' hostility. Maybe – as happens with primitives – a zero has been added, to mean 'many'. Even so, the situation fulfils one basic requirement of a plague: a large number of people travelling to strange lands where they have no acquired immunity to the endemic infections.

Whereas nomadic hunter-gatherers left their excrement behind them when they moved on, once people settled in villages in contact with other villages for trade by barter during the agricultural revolution and built more or less permanent homes, they had the problem of disposing of it safely. 'Safely' is the operative word. A polluted water supply or lack of clean water for washing hands still ensures the return of fecal matter to the food supply in many countries. An exhibit at the impressive Jorvik visitor centre of Scandinavian York, England is a coprolite stool, passed by some Viking inhabitant and excavated during the preparation of the underground visitor centre. Scientific analysis under the microscope revealed the presence of several species of intestinal worms, any one or all of which might carry even smaller and more dangerous parasites. The ubiquity of gastro-intestinal worms is such that, all over the world a very large number of mosses, lichens, weeds and tree-sap extracts have been used as vermifuges in deworming sufferers.

Another problem of early settlements, which still continues in many Third World countries, was the way inhabitants lived in close proximity to domesticated animals, which was a relatively new development in the history of the human race. A large number of diseases afflicting humans are shared with animals: poultry, 26; rats and mice, 32; horses, 35; pigs, 42; sheep and goats, 46; cattle, 50; dogs, 65.[12] Since some diseases are shared by several animal species, there is some overlap, but, clearly, living close to animals is dangerous. In Southeast Asian villages many families live for security reasons above their pigs and chickens with only a woven bamboo floor separating them, through which infected animals' exhalations easily pass while the owners are sleeping on the floor. In Africa, local wildlife is also a constant source of infection: bubonic plague and Lassa fever from rodents, rabies carried by bats, yellow fever and Ebola from monkeys eaten as 'bush meat', often undercooked. The list is long.

Gastro-intestinal worms were probably endemic in early settlements, as they are in the Third World today. More seriously, conditions were already ideal for epidemics of viral or bacterial infection. A gruesome proof of this was revealed by a team of archeologists from northeastern China's Jilin University working from 2011 to 2015 at a site called Hamin Mangha in southern Mongolia. They uncovered a village of twenty-nine houses half-sunk in the earth for protection against the harsh winter weather – a building technique still used today in Central Asia. They were mostly simple one-room structures containing a hearth, dating to approximately 5,000 years ago. In this well-ordered village with all houses spaced out and orientated in the same direction with their back to the prevailing winds, remains of stone pestles and mortars, digging tools, arrows, spear-heads and some jade jewellery testify to the mixed economy of a transitional Neolithic hunter-gatherer/farming population. They buried their dead and threw their rubbish into pits. They had also dug a defensive ditch around the village, with probably a palisade on the inner bank. This tells us that there were other humans nearby, from whom they were protecting themselves.

In one of these single-roomed dwellings measuring 14 feet by 15 feet, ninety-seven bodies of both sexes and all ages had been packed in on top of each other and the house destroyed by fire, making a common funeral pyre. At other Neolithic sites in the region more mass graves have been found, the bodies coming from people of all ages and both sexes. At Hamin Mangha the rest of the village showed no sign of being destroyed or damaged by armed attack. Since the making of stone tools is a difficult and time-consuming process, why did the inhabitants leave so many precious stone artifacts in good condition behind, instead of taking them along when they left? This now being a semi-desert region, the village was literally buried in the sands of time until the team from Jilin started digging. The only explanation for the precipitate abandonment of Hamin Mangha and the other contemporary villages excavated in the region with mass graves is an epidemic of a virulent killer disease.

Chapter 2

Of Cities and Armies

Once humans clustered in the assumed safety of increasingly large fortified towns and cities, seeking security from attacks by other humans, they created ideal conditions for pathogens to spread rapidly from person to person. This begs the question as to why the pathogens were ready and waiting for this moment, which will be addressed at the end of this book.

Hollywood's film sets of royal palaces and rich Roman and Greek families' villas give no idea of the reality of the cramped and insanitary conditions, lacking water and sanitation, in which the general populations lived in close contact with domestic animals and rodent parasites. At the same time, armies grew ever larger in order to attack the enemies' fortifications. From casual raids in search of plunder and slaves, organised warfare came into being and, as one ancient Chinese general commented, even a victorious army will lose many men to disease, simply because they are exposed to unfamiliar pathogens while on campaign in foreign parts. During the American war in Vietnam some 25,000 cases of plague were reported, most of the victims being indigenous people.[1]

In the conflict between Bronze Age Egypt and the Hittite empire, around 1274 BCE, a Hittite army of about 50,000 men, plus war horses and pack animals marched 1,000 miles south from the fortress-capital of Hattusha in modern Anatolia. Arriving at the southernmost tip of their empire, a city called Kadesh on the Orontes, which also marked the northernmost tip of Rameses II's Egyptian empire, they confronted the pharaoh's might. Both armies, strengthened by contingents from subject races, spearheaded their attacks with so many chariots that the combined number in the field was thought to be as high as 5,000, maybe more – which would make this the greatest chariot battle of all time.

It was a messy fight with both sides claiming the victory, not for the first or last time in military history. Afterwards the Hittites marched and rode back northwards to their impregnable fortress-city at Hattusha, with its five miles of defensive walls and towers at 60-foot intervals enclosing some 40,000 inhabitants. Archeologists exploring the ruins of Hattusha discovered five entire libraries of baked clay tablets written in a cuneiform script. When eventually deciphered, they were found to be the royal archives of the kingdom, covering laws, punishments, trade and military matters. There was even a copy of the peace treaty agreed with Ramses II after the battle of Kadesh – the earliest such document known.[2] All was constantly updated by the meticulous royal scribes. Yet, at some indeterminate time, Hattusha, built with a colossal investment of labour and time, was abandoned so fast that no mention of the reason has ever been found in all the libraries of clay tablets. Why?

In Egypt and Mesopotamia, in the absence of any scientific explanation, plagues were taken to be expressions of a god's anger. According to the Old Testament Book of Exodus,[3] at an undefined time the Hebrew leader Moses took advantage of this by threatening the reigning pharaoh with a series of ten plagues that his god Yahweh would inflict on Egypt if the Hebrew people were not freed and allowed to leave the land of the Nile. The Old Testament is not history and the story has been re-located by some scholars referring to the sixth-century BCE Babylonian exile of the Hebrews. Yahweh's ten pestilences included invasions of locusts, frogs and the like. Three, however, do sound like infectious diseases.

The fifth plague (Ex. 9:1-7) allegedly caused massive death of livestock. This could have been foot-and-mouth disease, caused by any one of seven viruses affecting cows, sheep, goats and other cloven-hoofed animals, becoming pandemic in Britain and other countries 1998–2001 and breaking out again in 2007. As with early humans, wild cattle in small herds might naturally recover from the effects, but in large herds of domesticated cattle under agricultural conditions, disease spreads very fast.

The sixth plague, which affected humans (Ex. 9:8-12) sounds somewhat like bubonic plague, when growths described as 'boils' appeared on victims' skin, but it might have been typhus. Or it could have been anthrax, which takes between one and five days to incubate in the human body, giving symptoms like the onset of a cold. Several days after infection, proliferating bacteria will be starting to engulf the lymph nodes and attack the lungs, filling them with liquid and preventing respiration, with choking fits and convulsions. Nine out of ten human victims die, if untreated.

The tenth plague (Ex. 1-12) was widespread child mortality. In the narrow Nile valley, bordered on both sides by uninhabitable desert, the population was densely concentrated, so that infection passed quickly from family to family and village to village. The situation continues today, especially in the Sahel or sub-Saharan Africa, where the likelihood of an infant dying is sixty times greater than that in developed Western countries.

Living several centuries BCE, Moses may have been claiming that regular outbreaks of disease among people and domestic animals were plagues sent by Yahweh. We simply do not know. However, many prehistoric civilisations from China to the Indus valley to Mesoamerica and South America died out very rapidly. The evidence is clear. Archeologists were for long baffled as to why, in the absence of any evidence of war, entire nations should have left their cities mysteriously undamaged and intact, as would not have been the case, had war driven out the population or killed them off. Virulent epidemics are the only feasible explanation.

Once writing was invented, evidence of epidemics becomes clear. In the fifth century BCE, the dramatist Sophocles described in his play *Oedipus Rex* a *thanatofora* or fatal disease in the city of Thebes whose unpleasant effects included causing women to miscarry or suffer stillbirths. Analysis by modern medical researchers has produced several possible pathogens, of which the most likely cause was *brucella abortus*, suggesting a zoonotic origin in cattle. Historian Thucydides described the plague of Athens in 429 BCE, the second year of the Peloponnesian war, when the city was besieged by the army of Sparta and its allies and the city was crammed with refugees from the fighting. Symptoms were severe headaches, inflamed eyes, sneezing, coughing blood, chest pains, vomiting and diarrhoea, small blisters and open sores on the skin. Unquenchable thirst with the fever drove some victims to throw themselves into open cisterns. Most became delirious and died a week or so after infection. Many of those who recovered had lost the use of limbs and suffered problems of memory and eyesight afterwards. The infection, Thucydides said, reached Athens from the port of Piraeus, brought by ships from Africa, and killed 25 per cent of the people sheltering within the walls, which would mean a death toll of 75,000-100,000 victims. Although he recovered from the infection, the Athenian general Pericles did not. The Spartans abandoned the siege from fear of contagion during the first outbreak, but carried this haemorrhagic fever back home with them anyway.

Plague reappeared in Athens in 427–26 BCE, but was it the same one? In 1994–95 CE excavations in the Athenian suburb of Karameikos at the site of a planned metro station revealed a large plague pit, from roughly this time.[4] Traces of *salmonella enterica serovar typhi* in three skeletons do not seem connected with this plague because this pathogen was already endemic in Greece, so it may have been smallpox, manifesting itself in pustular rashes, fever and diarrhoea. By the time of Sophocles and Thucydides, ever-larger cities, increasing international trade and frequent warfare produced the ideal conditions for this and other plagues. A city under siege, with many terrified refugees from the surrounding countryside crammed temporarily inside the walls with no proper sanitation, provided perfect conditions for incubation of infectious diseases to reach epidemic proportions.

Armies on campaign, as in the Peloponnesian war, also increased the spread of diseases even further, as repeatedly evidenced for 2,500 years into the twentieth century, with the misnamed Spanish 'flu pandemic, brought to Europe by shipments of US troops in 1918. President Woodrow Wilson was advised of the risk of moving many thousands of men who were suffering from a highly infectious and dangerous disease from training camps in Kansas and sending them across the Atlantic, but was swayed by the arguments of his generals in France, claiming that their urgent need of reinforcements, to replace the 58,000 casualties they had lost, outweighed the health risk, which they severely underestimated. Once the men were embarked on three-tier bunks aboard the commandeered passenger vessels serving as troopships, contagion was assured during the voyage. Many men were ill and some were already dying when they were disembarked in the French port of Brest. The total deaths of the pandemic this began are estimated by some sources as between 50 and 100 million.

The Roman historian and philosopher Titus Livius (64 BCE–12 CE) wrote a history entitled *Ab urbe condita* – from the foundation of the city. He mentions eleven plagues during the Republic, starting in 387 BCE. Rufus of Ephesus and Aretaeus of Cappadoccia, both famous Greek physicians writing about the beginning of the second century of the Common Era described the symptoms of a disease that sounds like bubonic plague.

In the second century CE, so great was the depopulation of some areas of the Roman Empire that barbarians, far from being held at bay on the fortified frontier known as the *limes*, were invited to come and settle on land that had previously been farmed by deceased Roman citizens. Half a century after Livy's death another plague struck, followed by the pandemic, possibly smallpox, that hit the empire in 165 CE. The Antonine plague was brought into the empire by troops returning from the siege of the city of Seleucia on the Tigris river in modern-day Iraq.[5] It is thought to have been smallpox. According to historian Dio Cassius, it killed one in four victims, accounting at its height for 2,000 deaths a day in Rome. Total of deaths during the pandemic has been estimated at 5 million, a third of the population in the countries affected.

Travelling with the legions – those self-contained armies – their own numbers much reduced by the infection, it reached furthest Gaul and the *limes* on the Rhine, where it evened the odds up to some extent by infecting also the invading barbarian tribes. Summoned to Rome, the Greek physician Galen (129–210 CE)[6] described the symptoms as fever, diarrhoea and sore throats with a skin eruption sometimes pustular appearing on the ninth day of infection. The most famous victim of this disease outbreak was the emperor Marcus Aurelius who, conscious of the risk of contagion, refused to see his son Commodus. When his sick father died seven days after infection, Commodus succeeded him. By then the plague – or plagues, if more than one disease was the cause of all the deaths – had been ravaging the Empire for fifteen years, suddenly to disappear and return nine years later.

At about the same time plague broke out in eastern China. Contact between the Roman and Chinese empires used to seem improbable, but Roman silverware, glass and coins, traded for silk and porcelain, have been found at archeological sites in Vietnam and China, tentatively dated to the early Han period (206 BCE–260 CE). A little known aspect of the silk trade is that, at Antioch before the Mediterranean stage of the long journey to Italy, the stout Chinese silken cloth was unravelled and re-woven into the semi-transparent material so sought by rich Roman ladies.[7] The re-working also had the commercial advantage that the middle-man sold more than he had bought.

In addition to the exchange of goods between the two widely separated empires along the old Silk Road, there was also some direct trade by sea routes. A Roman embassy to the Han Chinese court which set out in 166 CE were styled ambassadors of Emperor Marcus Aurelius, and criticised by one Chinese chronicler for bringing gifts less generous than would have been appropriate for His Celestial Majesty![8] How long these intrepid *gwailos* stayed is unknown, but the Chinese bureaucracy recorded a death rate of 30-40 per cent of tax-payers in an epidemic about then which began when the imperial army was fighting nomadic intrusions on the northwest frontier, so the Romans may have fled, carrying the infection back to Europe with them. Preceded by invasions of locusts and resultant famine, another Chinese plague occurred in 310–12 CE, which left alive only one or two out of 100 tax-paying inhabitants in the northwestern provinces, according to the next census. Ten years later, another plague spread far more widely – effectively a pandemic – killing *only* 2-3 per cent of the population. A Chinese doctor named Ho Kung (281–361 CE) recorded symptoms thus:

> Recently there have been persons suffering from epidemic sores which attack the head, face and trunk. In a short time, these sores spread all over the body. They have the appearance of hot boils containing some white matter. While some of these pustules are drying up, a fresh crop appears. If not treated early, the patients usually die. Those who recover are disfigured by purplish scars which do not fade until after a year.[9]

Was this smallpox? It seems likely, arriving in China at a time when the indigenous people would have no acquired immunity.

For several decades a Roman trading station for the commerce in spices was established on the Coromandel coast of southeastern India, south of modern Pondicherry. On the Veerampattinam peninsula Roman tiles, ostraca and footings of walls have been found, together with some jewels and coins. Also excavated were parts of Chinese-made screens and lacquered chests, indicating that the trading station also served as a halfway point for commerce with China. Traders there may have brought back to Europe a filovirus like Marburg fever or Ebola.

A documented plague of haemorrhagic fever first struck the eastern Roman empire centred on Constantinople in 249–62 CE and was probably the cause of joint-emperor Hostilian's death in November 251, although he may have been assassinated. When it reached Rome,

5,000 people died in the city each day. This pandemic was named the Cyprian plague after the Father of the Church and Bishop of Carthage Cyprian, who lived through the plague and described it in a detailed essay entitled *de mortalitate*:

> Constant diarrhoea weakens the whole body; swellings appear in the throat; the intestines are shaken with a continual vomiting; the eyes are on fire and blood-shot; in some cases the feet or parts of the lower limbs are lost through gangrene or the gait is enfeebled, the hearing obstructed, or sight impaired.[10]

The Christians were widely blamed for this plague, one of the victims of the consequent repression being Cyprian himself, martyred because he refused to give up his faith.

Dr Kyle Harper of the University of Oklahoma considered that this pandemic might even have contributed to the end of the Roman Empire as numerous usurpers of imperial power tried their luck in the civil and political chaos that it wrought. Also, the frontiers could not be adequately guarded due to many deaths in the legions, only the fortuitous contagion of the barbarian peoples pushing in on the borders saving the day. In 270 CE an outbreak of either the same or another plague killed off the militarily very successful emperor Claudius II Gothicus after a reign of only sixteen months.

A series of massive volcanic eruptions in the 530s and 540s CE caused climate change on a massive scale with temperatures dropping and downpours of rain. In the Northern hemisphere, as crops failed, the plague was waiting to take advantage of the weakened population of the Mediterranean basin. Byzantine emperor Justinian I (482–565 CE) caught bubonic plague in 541 CE. Although he recovered, some 25 million other victims around the inland sea died in this outbreak, including the great Byzantine general Belisarius (505–565 CE). Justinian's military secretary was the respected contemporary historian Procopius of Caesarea, who described his master's symptoms well: fever, delirium and buboes – the black swellings of the lymphatic glands in the armpits, behind the ears and in the groin, the last earning the name *pestis inguinariai* – plague in the groin. Most sufferers died, some still choking on the blood they were vomiting. This plague came from Egypt.

Justinian survived; one third of his subjects did not. The pandemic killed an estimated 25 million people in countries around the Mediterranean and changed the course of history. Procopius conveyed something of the incomprehension of the people of Byzantium:

> During these time there was a pestilence by which the whole human race came near to being annihilated. Now, in the case of all other scourges sent from heaven, some explanation of a cause might be given by those who are clever in these matters, for they love to conjure up causes which are absolutely incomprehensible to man. But, for this calamity it is quite impossible to express in words, or to conceive in thought any explanation, except indeed to refer it to God.[11]

In its first visit to Byzantium lasting four months, up to 10,000 people died in the city each day. Coping with burials on that scale was a major problem. The cause, some logical Greeks decided, was not the anger of a god, but infected fleas on rats which crawled ashore along the mooring ropes of merchant ships coming from Africa. Once ashore, after the rats died, their fleas transferred the bacillus to human hosts when injecting their blood-thinning saliva. Merchant ships carried the infection throughout the known world, the disease flaring up and dying down many times until 700 CE, by which year it is estimated that 50 per cent of the population of the Mediterranean countries had died. Arab sources record several outbreaks in the Middle East: in 627; again in 638; in Iraq during 688, 706, 716 and then every ten years or so until 744.[12]

Archeobotanical investigations in the Negev area of Israel found evidence of economic consequences of climate change at a number of sites, where a thriving viticultural area which had been exporting wine for more than 200 years suddenly gave up the production of *vinum gazetum* – a sweet white wine exported all over the Byzantine Empire through the port of Gaza. Farmers turned to growing wheat and barley for local consumption when the international wine market crashed.

In 580 CE Bishop Gregory of Tours recorded an epidemic in southern France characterised by pustules and tumours on the skin, which sounds more like smallpox than measles. Although now an endemic childhood disease, for which vaccination exists, the latter then frequently killed its victims of all ages. Originally, measles was not apparently a human disease but spilled over from cattle living in close proximity during the fourth century BCE.

Bubonic plague was first definitely recorded in China in 610 CE. But it was still around in 642, when a chronicler commented that it was rampant in the south near the port of Canton, eastern terminus of the maritime silk commerce, but rare in the interior. Something grave was happening in China in the early years of the Common Era. A tax census of the year 2 CE recorded 12.3 million hearths or dwellings in the kingdom; the census of 742 CE recorded only 8.9 million hearths. How much of this decline was due to epidemics and how much to war, is difficult to determine. When the Han dynasty died out in 220 CE, sixteen would-be successor states waged war and there was no central administration to hold back the barbarians in the northwest of the kingdom and the diseases they brought in with them.

Sino-American Professor of Far Eastern History Joseph H. Cha analysed Chinese documents compiled by local mandarins for the central administration in the capital listing human and natural calamities.[13] He listed 198 important epidemics in China between 16 CE and the year 1353, when the Black Death reached Europe. Many of these were caused by armies carrying infection to places where the inhabitants had no acquired immunity or where the soldiers had no immunity to locally endemic diseases.

In 16 CE a general attacking unnamed non-Chinese invaders 'in the south' lost between 60 and 70 per cent of his troops in this way. In 46 CE an epidemic associated with famine killed two-thirds of the population of Mongolia. In 162 CE an epidemic of plague in an army campaigning in Sinkiang and Kokonor killed 30 to 40 per cent of the soldiers. In 468 a pandemic killed hundreds of thousands of Chinese. In 762 more than half the population of Shantung province died. In 1227, half the population of Honan died and, in 1232 CE, 90,000 died from an epidemic there. The province of Hubei, where the 2019 coronavirus was first noted in the city of Wuhan, suffered confirmed plagues in 208, 468, 790, 891 and 1353 CE.[14]

For a long time, Japan's geographical and political isolation protected it from diseases on the Asian landmass. Thus, when there was contact, severe epidemics resulted. The first *recorded* contact with foreigners was in 552 CE, when Buddhist missionaries from Korea arrived, bearing their Indian philosophy – and smallpox, thought to have killed a million natives with no immunity. Later epidemics in 585, 698, 735, 763 and 790 were recorded, but in 808 CE what seems to have been bubonic plague from China killed half the population of the Japanese home islands. In 861, a disease named the coughing violence arrived and persisted for decades.

One of the problems of historians writing of the Dark Ages is that they lie in a period of renewed prehistory. As the Roman Empire neared its end and literacy went into European eclipse, a series of nomadic people pushed into the European Continent from the east, fleeing more aggressive peoples who had invaded their territory. Sometimes they fought the empire's soldiery; sometimes they fought with them against other newcomers. Their impact on the *pax romana* was cataclysmic. The period called the Great Migrations saw millions of people from ethnic groups including the Goths, the Vandals, the Alans or Alemanni and, of course, the Huns, sack the eternal city several times and turn it into the wasteland commented upon by medieval visitors: in 390 CE the Gauls under Brennus did the first damage; in 410 CE it was the Huns or Hiong-nu under Attila; in 455 the Vandals under Genseric; in 546 other Goths under Totila. As each wave of the barbarians arrived, it brought not just terror, bloodshed and destruction, but also new killer diseases.

Back in 444 CE there was a terrible epidemic in Britain, which changed our genetic inheritance. Their numbers depleted by famine and disease, the Britons called on the Saxons to help them fight the northern peoples with whom they were at war. These allies arrived in 449 and put the 'Saxon' into Anglo-Saxon. In what is now Austria the years 455 and 456 saw a mysterious disease that killed in three or four days. Even the Vandals, who had subjugated Spain and installed their own kingdom there and also sacked Rome in 455 CE, suffered both famine and plague that reduced their numbers in 478 or thereabouts. Earthquakes, tidal waves and volcanic eruptions wrought havoc and brought famine from Constantinople to Antioch, in which area three-quarters of a million people died from an epidemic of disease.

In the Indian sub-continent, smallpox seems – in the absence of any reliable records – to have installed itself early, with temples dedicated to a god of smallpox in the Hindu pantheon. The disease is caused by one of two *variola* viruses. Initial symptoms include fever and vomiting, followed by sores in the mouth and eruption of skin rashes, the spots turning into fluid-filled papules, whose scabs drop off, leaving disfiguring, lasting scars, with survivors often left blind. In some cases the skin lumps remain flat. The virulence of the highly infectious variola – one in three victims die – is such that it was estimated to have killed 300 million people in the twentieth century. The haemorrhagic form of the disease is characterised by bleeding into the skin, causing blackening, and earning the term *black smallpox*. Bleeding into the eyes turns the sclera – the white part of the eye – deep red and, invisibly but fatally, haemorrhages into the internal organs destroy them. The highly infectious nature of smallpox enabled European empire-builders to use it in biological warfare against indigenous peoples of both hemispheres, by giving them 'presents' of blankets or clothing that had been used by dead victims.

A Gloucestershire doctor, Edward Jenner noticed in 1796 that milkmaids who had contracted the similar but far milder cowpox from handling the pox-covered udders of cows they milked did not subsequently fall victim to smallpox. And what about the consumers of the infected cows' milk? Was it a prophylactic? We don't know. What we do know is that, after taking pus from a milkmaid's cowpox swelling, he scratched the skin on the arm of an 8-year-old boy called James Phipps and rubbed in some of the pus. Young Phipps eventually developed a scab at the site and had a mild fever. About six weeks later, Jenner took the risk of vaccinating the boy with smallpox virus. After being observed for several months, Phipps still had no reaction to it. Although Jenner was not the first person to conceive the notion of cowpox protecting against the smallpox virus, his experiment proved the theory. It was later discovered that the cowpox vaccination only worked temporarily against the invasion of smallpox and the procedure would need to be repeated several times through the patient's lifetime. Jenner named his technique *vaccination*, from the Latin for a cow: *vacca*. However, many more millions were to die before worldwide programmes of vaccination enabled the World Health Organisation to announce the global eradication of smallpox in 1980.

Although Jenner had the main claim to fame because he made vaccination a medical procedure in Britain and New England, a number of people who had contacts with cows had already used their powers of observation and logical deduction to test the possibility that cowpox vaccine could immunise humans against smallpox. In Dorset, England, one of them was a farmer named Benjamin Jesty who made the experiment in 1774. In 1791 a German schoolteacher named Peter Plett took a chance and inoculated his wife and two young sons with pus from a milkmaid's cowpox pustule, saving them from a smallpox epidemic in their town, then went on to save a number of other people in the same way. So it is possible that Dr Jenner had heard of these successful experiments, or others, for in parts of the Ottoman Empire, it seems, inoculation had been practiced for a century or more. In 1714, a letter written by Emanuel Timonius at Constantinople was read to the Royal Society by John Woodward:

> the writer of this ingenious discourse observed, in the first place, that the Circassians, Georgians and other Asiatics, had introduced the practice of 'procuring the smallpox' by a sort of inoculation among the Turks and others at Constantinople, and that although at first the more prudent were very cautious in the use of this practice; yet the happy success it has found to have in thousands of subjects, has put it out of all suspicion and doubt; since the operation, having been performed on persons of all ages, sexes, and different temperaments ... none have been found to die of the smallpox. They that have this inoculation practised upon them are subject to very slight symptoms, some being scarce sensible they are ill or sick: and what is valued by the fair, it never leaves and scars or pits in the face.

When this was published in the Philosophical Transactions of the Royal Society it triggered a reply from Cotton Mather, a minister in Boston, Massachusetts.

> I am willing to confirm to you, in a favourable opinion, of Dr. Timonius' communication; and therefore, I do assure you, that many months before I met with any intimations of treating the smallpox with the method of inoculation, anywhere in Europe; I had from a servant of my own an account of its being practised in Africa. Enquiring of my Negro man, Onesimus, who is a pretty intelligent fellow, whether he had ever had the smallpox, he answered, both

yes and no; and then told me that he had undergone an operation, which had given him something of the smallpox and would forever preserve him from it; adding that it was often used among the Guramantese [Libyans] and whoever had the courage to use it was forever free of the fear of contagion. He described the operation to me, and showed me in his arm the scar which it had left upon him; and his description of it made it the same that afterwards I found related unto you by your Timonius.

Mather said that he had had this conversation with Onesimus many months before he read the Timonius report, and his comments were confirmed by another minister who had talked with several slaves who had also been inoculated in Africa. In 1716 a physician named Jacob Pylarinius, also reported from Constantinople that inoculation had been introduced there by a Greek woman about 1660. It had been widely used by poor Christians until, during a severe smallpox epidemic in 1700, the practice spread throughout the Christian community more generally. But this was not inoculation with cowpox: the medium used was matter squeezed from a pustule of a person with smallpox. Yet, Lady Mary Wortley Montague, wife of the British ambassador to the Sublime Porte in Constantinople, discovered that variolation, as she called it, was widely practised in Turkey and considered so safe that she had had her son and daughter inoculated.

Two Welsh doctors wrote that variolation had been a common practice around the port of Haverfordwest since at least 1600. An English doctor living in Aleppo found that it was widely used around the Mediterranean, except by Muslims, who thought it against the will of God. As to how the practice had arrived in the Ottoman Empire, there were various conflicting reports: some believed it had come from India; others that it had come from China. By the early nineteenth century, more than 100,000 people in Great Britain and New England had been vaccinated: an amazing leap in public heath practice in less than one century.[15]

In 1790, British army medical officers investigated a belief in the military that mounted troops were less at risk from smallpox than the infantry were, due to their exposure to the similar horsepox virus, medical name *variola equina,* and found it was true. After a daughter of Spanish King Carlos IV (r. 1788–1808) caught smallpox in 1798 and was saved by Jenner's vaccination technique, the king had the entire royal family vaccinated and ordered his physician Francis Xavier de Balmis to distribute it throughout the then vast Spanish empire in North and South America. The problem was how to keep the vaccine fresh. From Spanish orphanages, de Balmis conscripted twenty-two boys aged from 3 to 9 years, who had never had smallpox. He vaccinated two of them at the start of the voyage and used the pus that appeared in the pustules on their arms to vaccinate two more – and so on until the end of the transatlantic voyage.

Many times and in many places, plagues changed the course of history, weakening the Byzantine and Roman garrisons along the Mediterranean littoral so that the Rashinun and Umayyad caliphates invading in 629 CE launched a ding-dong contest of faiths that lasted more than four centuries, including the First Crusade. In 732 CE the Moorish invaders reached as far north as Poitiers – a week's march from Paris – before Charles Martel drove them back across the Pyrenees, where they continued to occupy much of Spain, being slowly pushed back by the Reconquista, which lasted until 1492.

At the beginning of this period there was an unrelated epidemic after the Synod of Whitby attended by churchmen from England, Wales and Ireland in 664. It killed many thousands, including the archbishop of Canterbury and the bishop of London, and significantly depopulated southern coastal regions of England. Forty-eight other epidemics were reported by Anglo-Saxon sources between 526 and 1087 CE. Many seem to have weakened in the course of time, following the pattern by which tolerance builds up in the exposed population, leaving a disease that began by killing all ages to settle into a pattern of endemic, less harmful, childhood disease, as has happened with measles, mumps and other unpleasantnesses. There is evidence that in 569–80 and 986–88 there were contagious and fatal diseases shared by cattle and humans. This was in Europe's Dark Ages, so there is very little documentation. When King Alfred was king of the Anglo-Saxons (r. 886–899) there was an epidemic of what was called plague in 896. Exactly what it was, we don't know. At the time Alfred was engaged in all-out war against the armies of the Danelaw, fought in the main by roving bands of armed men burning crops, cutting down fruit trees, destroying dwellings and killing people and domestic animals – or driving the latter off as spoils of war. In such conditions, tens of thousands of people must have been starving or nearly so, making them easy prey for any rampant virus or bacterium. The latter word comes from the Greek *baktērion,* a diminutive of *baktron*, a rod – a reference to the rodlike shape of the pathogen under magnification.

In about 1,000 CE the human disease of measles – caused by the morbillivirus – split away from the bovine disease known as rinderpest, but before then during the periods above a similar but now-extinct morbillivirus infected both cattle and humans with fatal results for both species.[16]

In 1031 CE plague once again attacked the Indian sub-continent, coming from Central Asia with the army of Sultan Mahmud of Gazna. Another outbreak in 1403 reputedly destroyed the invading army of Sultan Ahmed in Malwa. The Mughal emperor Jahangir reported in 1619 that plague had been prevalent for three years in Agra, with about 100 people dying each day. He too described buboes in the armpits and groin, or at the base of the neck. There was a belief at the time that it was an affliction of the winter that disappeared in the heat of summer. These are just vague accounts, but in 1689 the Arabic historian Khafi Khan described the plague that had been ravaging the province of Dakhin and spread to Bijapur. His details are convincing: swellings as big as a banana under the arms, behind the ears, and in the groin.

War is the plague's great ally. In 1098 CE a Christian European army of the First Crusade about 300,000 strong besieged Antioch. So many died in the siege camps outside the walls that there were not enough survivors to bury them all, and the death of 5,000 of the 7,000 horses shipped out from Europe rendered the cavalry impotent. After the capture of Jerusalem in the following year only 60,000 crusaders were still alive – and their number dwindled to 20,000 by 1101.[16]

Chapter 3

What Makes a Pandemic?

Massive annual pilgrimages with the commensurate sanitation problems and close proximity of hundreds of thousands of people keep cholera alive in India. On a lesser, but still mortal scale, throughout the Middle Ages pilgrimages to Santiago de Compostela brought thousands of pilgrims through southwest France each summer. On the outward journey they used a pierced cockle shell carried on a leather thong around the neck, to scoop up drinking water from the streams they crossed. Since they were heading for the shrine of St Iago (Yakov originally in Hebrew, Jacques in French and James in English) at Compostela, this originated the gourmet seafood dish known as Coquilles St Jacques. On the return journey, they brought from Spain an innovation unknown in Northern Europe: stoppers for their water flasks made from the bark of the cork tree. But, like invading armies, they also brought with them diseases that killed the locals. Recent building work at a medieval church near the author's home in southwest France revealed a plague pit with dozens of skeletons all piled in from that period.

When Christopher Columbus 'discovered' the Caribbean islands in 1493, they were named for the anthropophagic Carib natives who inhabited them, sometimes referred to as *canibales*, which gave the English language a name for humans who eat their own kind. The neighbouring natives on the mainland, called Arawaks, seem to have lived in a state of intermittent warfare with the Caribs. Both races were enslaved to work in the mines when the Europeans discovered gold on Hispaniola. This atrocity paled into insignificance when Hernan Cortés' *conquistadores* landed on the mainland of Mexico in 1519 and destroyed the Aztec civilisation by, perhaps unintentional, biological warfare. The European diseases they brought, particularly smallpox, had been endemic in Europe for many centuries, killing around 30 per cent of victims and leaving the others with pockmarked scars. But in Aztec Mexico the arrival of the pox among people with no resistance to it

25

wiped out more than 10 million of the pre-conquest native population of 11 million, making the *conquistadores'* subjugation of Central and later South America easy. No women had accompanied Cortes' soldiers, who took their pleasure in raping or 'marrying' native women, some of whom had a posthumous revenge in having bestowed syphilis on their masters, which they brought back to Europe on their return.

A plague that struck Europe in the mid-fourteenth century was thought to have originated in the Orient, but this was not positively identified as the cause until a team of epidemiologists visited Manchuria to investigate a killer epidemic in 1921–24 and found a reservoir of bubonic plague in burrowing rodents of several species native to Central Asia, which apparently migrate from time to time due to climate change or earthquakes. Indeed, their presence in Central Asia is due to climate change. They originally came from the Qanghai-Tibetan plateau, but migrated south to warmer climes when the tectonic forces that elevated the Himalayas also raised the plateau to a height of 4,500 metres or nearly 15,000 feet.

Dendrochronology has revealed that the two years before the plague of Justinian (known in England as 'the plague of Cadwalader's time') and the two years before the first Black Death were extremely cold throughout Eurasia. Earthquakes also disturbed the underground cities of these rodents, which decamped *en masse* to new territory. It was already known from Russian investigations in the Don-Volga region that rodent species there carried the plague, although this did not necessarily mean that they were the vectors by which plague reached humans.[1]

Bubonic plague reached China's Hubei Province in 1353. That plague had also travelled west with merchants' caravans along the Great Silk Road.[2] These caravans stopped for the night in caravansarais, within the walls of which they would be safe from robbers. Locally infected fleas also established themselves in the caravansarais and, since fleas can live for months without a blood meal, they were happy to install themselves in the camels' loads or saddle bags and get a free trip to the western terminal of the Silk Road.

War also played a part: in 1347 CE the Mongols in their second invasion of Europe used biological warfare, catapulting corpses of plague victims over the walls of the besieged Crimean city of Kaffa, modern Feodosiya in Ukraine. There was nothing new about this tactic. During the period of the crusades (1095–1492), both Christian and

Muslim besiegers routinely used their siege engines to hurl diseased and rotting human and animal carcases into cities under attack. What makes the gruesome tactic even more horrible is that prisoners taken in a sortie were used to clean up the mess, so that they, and not the defenders, would catch any infection it contained.

Kaffa had been a shantytown inhabited by fisherfolk in 1266 when the foreign traders first arrived to take advantage of its geographical position. Eighty years later, commercial development had made a port that could hold 200 ships and a town encircled with double walls that boasted 6,000 houses within the inner walls and another 5,000 between the inner and outer walls, accommodating altogether as many as 80,000 inhabitants. Spreading up the crescent of slopes above the town were the luxurious villas of rich foreign merchants, whose fortunes had been made by trade in silks from the East and timber from the far North floated down the Don, Volga and Dnieper rivers. Ukrainian slaves were also bought and sold. Negotiations were conducted in a score of languages.

Merchants coming from the East brought news of terrible disasters in China – of locusts eating all the crops and causing starvation, of floods carrying away thousands of people and earthquakes that swallowed whole towns and even a mountain. A mysterious disease killed off 5 million people. To these more or less factual rumours, in the manner of the time were added horrific details – frogs, lizards, scorpions and fire raining down from Heaven, and destructive tempests that lasted days on end with enormous hail stones flattening crops and destroying houses.[3]

The mainly Italian foreign traders were protected in Kaffa by a treaty with the Tartars, but there were sporadic tensions. The final straw was a riot in 1343 that broke out in Tana, a city at the mouth of the Don whence the trans-Asia caravans departed for the eight-month trek to China, which often took even longer because of foul weather en route. The killing in the riot of a Muslim Tatar prompted a Mongol khan named Janibeg to declare war on the Christians in Tana. Whether diplomacy could have saved the day, who can say? Instead, their insolent reply to his ultimatum triggered the unleashing of hundreds of his mounted warriors on the town. Breaking in, they drove the Italian merchants, literally with fire and sword, down to the harbour, where they hastily weighed anchor and set out to sea, heading for Kaffa. The voyage of 400 miles the whole length of the Sea of Azov and through the strait of Kerch into the Black Sea did not provide the hoped-for safety. Soon after the Genoese arrived in Kaffa, the Mongol horde arrived by land and camped in the hills above the city. The richer merchants abandoned their luxury villas and sought protection inside the city walls.

The real enemy was not mounted on a shaggy steppe pony. In 1333 a terrible drought had caused widespread famine in China, exacerbated by swarms of locusts consuming what crops had been grown. Simultaneously, earthquakes and floods in the following years killed many, causing a death toll estimated at many millions. In these conditions, ideal for plague, it spread like wildfire and, as survivors fled westwards towards what they hoped would be better conditions, they carried the plague with them, infecting India and Persia and reaching Tatary and the Crimea. According to Ibn al-Wardi, a contemporary chronicler in Aleppo,[4] this fatal progress took years. Some respite was afforded to Kaffa by an Italian relief force that arrived in 1344 and drove the Mongols off with heavy losses. By 1346 it had reached the western shores of the Caspian Sea and travelled up the Akhtuba river to Sarai Batu, where the Golden Horde was headquartered, financed by the profits from the largest slave market in Europe or Asia.

A year later, it had crossed the Don and Volga rivers and made inroads into the Tatar siege camp at Kaffa. At first, the Christians inside the walls told themselves this was a miraculous salvation sent by God, but when cases of plague also began inside the city – whether or not due to infected corpses being catapulted over the walls – the Genoese traders living there fled homeward, thinking to save themselves. Briefly visiting Pera on the Black Sea, they continued on to Constantinople on the Bosphorus, where they infected the inhabitants, including the 13-year-old son of Emperor John VI Katakouzenos, who died. The grieving father wrote a treatise attributing the spread of the disease to merchant shipping. The royal archivist Nicephoras Gregoras described the mounting death toll, the uselessness of any available medicine and the panic of the population. He also mentioned that domestic animals like dogs and horses succumbed. Although this outbreak subsided after a year, plague returned to Constantinople ten times before 1400 CE and sixty-eight times in the eighteenth century.

In autumn 1347, carried reputedly on a slave ship from Constantinople,[5] plague reached Alexandria in Egypt. A year later, it was in Mecca, brought by pilgrims on the *hajj* and in Cairo, the largest city in the Mediterranean basin, whence the child sultan fled, leaving

600,000 of his subjects to die.[6] The plague was to return to Cairo more than fifty times in the next 150 years. From the border city of Gaza, the plague infected the whole of modern Syria, Lebanon, Israel and Iraq. The countries south of the Mediterranean were also all infected by 1349. Moving westward from Alexandria, plague spread through Libya to Tunisia, where the capital city was being besieged by a Moroccan army. Siege abandoned, the Moroccans carried the fatal bacillus home with them, where it met the plague arriving from Almeria in southern Spain[7] – at which point the whole Mediterranean basin was in the fatal embrace of the pandemic. Symptoms were fever, headaches, aching joints as in a bad influenza attack and the vomiting of blood. The second pandemic of plague raged somewhere in the Islamic world every year between 1500 and 1850,[8] and killed 1 million people in France, 1.7 million in Italy and 1.25 million in Spain.

Plagues, as the epitome of evil, find their way into many novels: Albert Camus' *La peste* is set in an outbreak of bubonic plague in French Algeria where its main character Dr Rieu does his best to fight it. All three of the tragic Brontë sisters used epidemic disease like the cholera of 1848–49 in their books. *Love in the Time of Cholera* by Gabriel García Márquez and *Death in Venice* by Thomas Mann have cholera as the terrifying background to the plots. Olivia Manning's *Balkan Trilogy* has its heroine Harriet Pringle and a woman friend finding themselves the sole guests in a remote Egyptian hotel because all the other clients have rightly fled from a local cholera outbreak. Yet, the most famous plague-inspired book is Giovanni Boccaccio's *The Decameron* – a collection of fourteenth-century tales told by seven young women and three men escaping the plague in Florence by fleeing the city to take refuge in a country house. Boccaccio described the sequence well:

> [Plague] first betrayed itself by the emergence of tumours in the groin or armpits, some of which grew as large as apples, others like eggs, which the common folk called *gavoccioli*. These began to spread all over, after which black or livid spots showed on the arms or legs. The *gavoccioli* and these spots were a certain sign of approaching death.[9]

Some victims recovered from the bubonic form, but very few survived the pneumonic form of the disease, which attacked the lungs and respiratory apparatus or the more rare septicaemic form, which killed so fast that, within hours, the victim's blood swarmed with plague bacilli, giving the buboes no time to appear before death.[10] During one outbreak in the early twentieth century, average survival time from infection to death was 14.5 hours.[11]

As historian John Kelly asks, how did the ships from Kaffa with plague-infected crews manage to make a successful voyage lasting several months?[12] Were some of the men naturally immune? Would new crew members sign on at intermediate ports, to work alongside terminally sick seamen? A monk in Messina named Friar Michele described the symptoms of those on the ship, from which it is obvious that the infection in his home town manifested itself as droplet-born pneumonic plague. Somehow or other, the twelve Genoan galleys from Kaffa carried the pathogen to Sicily and Italy with them, transiting via numerous ports *en route* including Ragusa (modern Dubrovnik in Croatia, which was then a Venetian possession), where the city council passed a law as early as 1377 headed *veniens de locis pestiferis non intret Ragusium vel districtum* – 'Anyone coming from plague-infected places may not enter Ragusa city or district.' There were strict punishments and fines for defying the quarantine period of thirty days (*il trentino*).

In 1448, so many citizens fled the plague-threatened city of Venice that the senate informed city employees that they must return to their posts within a week or lose their jobs. The senate also extended the period of isolation to forty days (*il quarantino*)[13] and took over the islands of San Giorgio d'Alega and San Marco Boccacalame in the lagoon as quarantine areas for new arrivals. But still the deaths mounted up to 600 in a single day, making an estimated total of 72,000 people. The period of forty days was thought to be particularly efficacious because it was the length of time Christ was believed to have spent in the wilderness. A record of the precipitate flight of the Genoese traders from Kaffa and their return to Italy was kept by Gabriele de' Mussis, a notary in Piacenza whose profession it was to keep meticulous notes of wills and inheritances.

Not called Black Death at the time, but referred to simply as 'the pestilence' – from the Latin *pestilentia* – the plague bacillus raced around the continent of Europe clockwise from port to port, carried by *mus rattus* – the black rats on board trading ships. Navigation at the time was by portolan maps, the merchant ships staying as close to land as possible as they swung from one port to the next. This practice avoided being caught in the open sea when the weather changed, which was often fatal for the round-bottom ships of the period – as the annual crop of wrecks in the Mediterranean explored by modern submarine archeology bears out.

However, at each port of call, plague spread into the interior, morbidity varying widely up to 100 per cent of victims, partly because a series of wet and cold summers 1315–22 had produced famine throughout much of Europe, lowering the resistance of the victims. In England, famines had killed hundreds of thousands in 1272, 1277, 1283, 1292 and 1311, arguably with the benefit of reducing a previous over-population, general throughout Europe. At the same time, with crop yields for medieval species of grain often little better than two grains harvested for each one planted and commoners eating little meat, all it took was two or more consecutive wet summers to leave the general population starving and weak even before an epidemic struck. If the nobility at first suffered less in times of famine, they were still not immune to contagion from the infected lower orders on their estates.

From the port of Pisa, the plague leapt inland to Florence, where measures to reduce the population of rats also saw prostitutes and homosexuals expelled as being possible targets for divine punishment. In the city, free bread was distributed to 94,000 people who could show tickets of entitlement; repayments of debts were suspended; prison gates were thrown open to all except the most dangerous criminals. These measures did not stop a huge earthquake devastating northern Italy. Church bells were silenced and the wearing of mourning clothes forbidden as being too depressing for those still healthy. Denial was rampant, many wealthier citizens forming ten-man dining clubs, despite the numbers attending declining nightly as plague struck one after another. In San Gimignano, 58 per cent of the inhabitants died; in Siena and Orvieta almost as many. The chronicler of Este alleged that 63,000 died in and around Naples

A bankrupted Florentine banker, Giovanni Villani described the progression of the plague, attributing it to sinister astrological conjunctions. Dishonest officials reputedly stole 375,000 gold florins from estates of the dead. Was this why the chief of the Florentine police was forced to witness the execution and dismemberment of his son before himself receiving the same treatment?[14] The collapse of great banks is not a modern phenomenon: the Peruzzi went bankrupt in 1343; the Acciaiuoli and the Bardi followed in 1345; the Florentine banks had lost 1.7 million florins. And war – that great midwife of epidemics – tore the country to pieces, with the pro-German Ghibellines fighting the pro-Pope Guelphs, the Orsini and the Colonna families (each of which had furnished the Church with many cardinals and several popes) fighting each other and the Visconti family of Milan fighting everybody. Whilst the knightly class and men at arms profited from this strife, the general population suffered and starved.

When plague reached Rome in August 1348 Pope Clement VI declared it was divine punishment for mankind's sins, but he was far away in his palatial exile at Avignon. There, people refused to eat fish, which they thought were contaminated by infected air, and spices too, for fear lest they had been transported to Europe on Genoese galleys. They indulged in hysterical candlelight processions at night, some beating, or flagellating, themselves with whips until the blood flowed. They lit bonfires to clean the air and also burned Jews until Clement issued a bull denouncing this as murder. He also promised the remission of sins for all who died of the plague.[15] The greatest nobility was shown by monks at the municipal almshouse, who cared for and treated the plague-stricken with no thought for their own contagion.[16] It is easy in reading all the bewildering statistics to overlook that most of the millions of deaths were tragedies for grieving parents, children and friends. When, after years of unrequited love, the poet Francesco Petrarca, anglicised as Petrarch, lost his beloved Laura in 1348, he wrote that 'death looked lovely in her face'. But this is poetic licence: nobody dying of the plague looked lovely and instinct told the survivors to get rid of the corpse by any means, fast, for fear of contagion. It is most unlikely that he saw her corpse.

Although mysteriously missing some territories in the Welsh and Irish mountains and the high Pyrenees, the Low Countries and the Polish marshes, probably because people living there had little or no contact with outsiders, the clockwise progress of the plague around Europe was so rapid that it reached Russia five or six years later; its complementary vectors being shipborne black rats and the fleas they carried. Modern DNA research indicates that the black rat did not originate in Europe, but southern India. Since traces of it have been found in England as far back as Norman times, it may have taken advantage of Roman-era maritime routes from Pondicherry back to Rome and through the empire to cover most of Europe.

The species *mus rattus* is an efficient vector for several diseases, due to its ability to tolerate many bacteria in its bloodstream. These, sucked up by rat fleas designated *Xenopsylla cheopsis*, infect the fleas, which in turn pass the infection on to their new hosts when a rat dies from the infection or otherwise. It has been hazarded that the eventual decline of the Black Death was due to the smaller but more cold-tolerant grey rat designated *rattus norvegicus* gradually replacing black rats in Europe, but that did not happen until the eighteenth century, so the chronology is wrong. In any case, many experts have cast doubt on a rat-borne plague being able to travel so fast across and round Europe. Scientists at the Public Health England infectious diseases lab at Porton Down maintain that for the plague to spread so far so fast also required a pneumonic form of the microbe, spread faster by coughs and sneezes than the rat-flea vector could have achieved.

Estimates of total fatalities vary in the range 75 million to 200 million in Europe, Africa and Asia. American medievalist Philip Daileader considers it likely that this plague killed off 45 per cent or more of the European population;[17] Norwegian historian Ole J. Bendictow estimated the fatalities as being higher.[18] The percentages of women and children killed were higher, possibly because they spent more time indoors where the risk of infection by flea-bite was more acute. The dying convulsions of infected pregnant women invariably caused them to expel the foetus, whatever its stage of development.

Chapter 4

Research and Regulations

Epidemiology is a modern science, but before it existed formally there were a few physicians and philosophers who tried to figure out how diseases could travel both far and fast. A Veronese physician and polymath called Girolamo Fracastro (1476–1563) rejected Galen's theory of miasmas and proposed that disease was caused by particles or life-forms too small to see at the time, which was a spot-on guess. Fracastro's book *de contagion et contagiosis morbis* was on the right track, particularly in suggesting that better personal hygiene could be useful to keep infection at bay.

At the time, plague was hitting Scotland, where sufferers were isolated to three islands in the Firth of Forth: Inch Keith, Inch Colm and Inch Garvie. The last name was derived from the Gaelic words *Innis Garbhach* meaning 'the rough island'. Given the exposed nature of these small islands and the often foul weather of the Forth, it would seem that these destinations were intended as comfortless waiting rooms for death. In another outbreak a century later during 1568–69, similar treatment awaited the 2,500 plague victims in Edinburgh, who suffered fainting fits, sweating, vomiting, bloody dark urine, cramps, convulsions, colic, dropsy-like swelling of the body and other unpleasant symptoms. Their clothes were taken away and boiled and they were cast out of the city, to live in makeshift hovels on the moors and die there.

Dr Thomas Sydenham (1624–1689) analysed Fracastro's detailed and methodical notes on his patients and their symptoms to classify diseases, but was prevented by his Puritan beliefs from practising any autopsies. Yet, his book *Observationes medicae* was used as a textbook for more than a century. Although he identified the condition called St Vitus' Dance, caused by a streptococcus bacterium, his greatest frustration was being unable to identify the cause of smallpox. John Graunt (1620–1674) was a wealthy haberdasher with an interest in statistics. His tabulation of the Bills of Mortality (see below) refuted some unfounded beliefs about disease and supported several new ones.

Even before these original thinkers, Magister Raimundus, employed by the exiled pope in Avignon, composed a treatise entitled *De epidemica*, in which he noted soberly that in 1347–48 two-thirds of the population there became infected and most of them died. Among the victims of this plague were all five children of Sienese chronicler Agnolo di Tura, who had to bury them with his own hands.[1] In 1362 Raimundus recorded that half the population of Europe was infected but deaths were fewer proportionately. In 1371 one tenth was infected, with many surviving. In 1382, it mainly affected children.

Nearly two millennia earlier, Hippocrates had studied and written about epidemics, introducing several principles of what would be known as epidemiology. He asserted that the incidence of epidemics can be related to variations in the weather and living conditions, with people's habits, diet and activity all playing their parts. Including the disease prognosis of several patients to support his theories in the book, this was the first medical work to present case series, as in a modern report. For most cases, he mentioned age, gender, place of residence and the seasonal conditions at the time of onset of the illness. He also described the symptoms, noting morbidity and mortality, modes of transmission of infectious diseases, and took into account what might be termed genetic vulnerability, e.g. a woman who had a 'congenital tendency to phthisis'. Such a word has to be Greek! It meant a wasting disease, later termed consumption and now tuberculosis, which is reckoned to have killed one in seven of all humans from prehistory to the nineteenth century. Hippocrates condemned intemperance in drinking, overeating and sexual excess. In another work he postulated that diseases should be studied in light of the season in which they happen, so that a good physician could predict likely seasonal waves of illness, distinguishing between endemic sickness and epidemics. His wide spread of knowledge included many disciplines including urology, proctology, gynecology, pediatrics and even dermatology.

Yet no developments in the historic West continued building on this solid foundation. In the East, however, Arabic scientists embraced the wisdom of Greek and Roman sources. Ibn an-Nafis (1210–1288) was a Damascene physician who practised also in Cairo, making his own discoveries in the fields of cardiology and pulmonary blood circulation.

He also profited from translations of Hippocrates' and Galen's works, and used writings by his Islamic predecessors like Ibn al-Rhazi, known in the West as Rhazes.[2] Among Westerners whose lives were saved while in the Orient during the crusades were King Philippe Auguste of France and England's Richard the Lionheart.

How much or how little of this precious knowledge seeped through to the West, is hard to say. Practising as both physician and surgeon, Raimundus freely admitted that the common medieval practice of bleeding the sick had no effect, although he continued to prescribe it for priests he did not like – presumably to stop them complaining to Pope Clement that he had refused to treat them. Some barber-surgeons cut into any accessible vein when bleeding a patient; others used a pseudo-science, according to which certain veins functioned as emunctories – cleansing or excretory ducts for the organs of the body – that of the heart being in the armpit and that of the liver in the groin. There was more logic in cutting open the buboes to release the pus and sepsis within. Ibn Khatimah (1323?–1369), a Moorish physician practising in Almeria, believed the time to do this was between the third and seventh day of infection. There was a *caveat*: he warned that a mistake in timing resulted in death of the patient anyway.

Where Raimundus was wildly wrong was in attributing the plague to unfavourable astronomical conjunctions, but in this he was not alone: the considered opinion of the doctors in the medical faculty of Paris, given to King Philippe VI de Valois when the plague arrived there in May or June of 1348 – lasting until the winter of 1349 – was that an unfavourable conjunction of three planets had caused fatally poisonous miasmas.[3] The big advantage, of course, in subscribing to this theory, or pretending to, was that only God could control the movement of heavenly bodies, so no mortal was to blame if he failed to find a cure. When King Philippe left Paris for the north in August, the disease followed him into Normandy. Every *savant* weighed in with his opinion, not always disinterestedly. At the University of Montpellier in southern France the teacher Alfonso de Cordoba opined that the plague was caused by

> an eclipse of the moon occurring immediately before in the sign of Leo accompanied by a powerful alignment of unlucky planets. The best remedy is to flee the plague and the use of pestilential pills that I manufacture is of great value.

36

A more rational German master of philosophy and theology who had taught in the Paris schools, Conradus Megenburgensis (1309–1374) pointed out that no astronomical conjunction lasted longer than two years; since some plagues did last longer, they could not have been caused by a conjunction of planets.

Some thinkers recalled the idea of matter being composed of tiny particles, as first proposed by Epicurus (341–270 BCE). He wrote that you could cut anything smaller and smaller until you reached the *atomos* – the uncuttable atom or ultimate particle. The Roman poet Lucretius (99–55 BCE) reworked this in his treatise entitled *de rerum natura* – concerning the nature of matter. Simple lenses for reading spectacles had surprisingly been around since the thirteenth century, to the great relief of monks copying books in their scriptoria, but the idea of aligning an objective lens near the object and an eyepiece a short distance away to magnify the object took a long time to develop. The invention is claimed by many different people. Almost certainly, it happened in the Netherlands, which had an advanced optical industry.

It could have been invented by Zacharias Janssen (1585–1632?) or his father. Another contender was Hans Lipperhey (1570–1619), who did apply for the first telescope patent in 1608. Cornelis Drebbel, another lens grinder who moved from the Netherlands to England is probably the true inventor, since he was known to have had one in London around 1619, but we do not know the magnifying power of these early instruments or how clear the images were in the eyepiece. Because of his fame for other inventions, even Galileo Galilei has been suggested as the inventor, but he was inspired by seeing a microscope made by Drebbel exhibited before the Accademia dei Lincei (the academy of the lynx-eyed) at Rome in 1624. Johann Faber (1574–1629), a German physician in Rome coined for it the name *microscope*, literally 'looking at small things'.

Just before the Great Plague in 1665 Robert Hooke's book *Micrographia* was published with shatteringly precise drawings of fleas and other small creatures. But the microscope really took off as a scientific instrument when Anton van Leeuwenhoek (1632–1723) in the Dutch town of Delft perfected a superior method of grinding lenses that produced an amazing 300x magnification with a single glass ball lens held between two metal plates. It did not look like a modern compound microscope, but did enable him to report on 9 October 1675 to the London Royal Society, of which he was a member, that, using this device he had been able to see red blood cells, spermatozoa and bacteria in bodily fluids. Unfortunately that instrument was not available to examine the matter taken from buboes or samples of victims' blood during the great plague, so theories about planetary conjunctions and miasmas continued.

As to the idea that Jews, for example, had sprinkled poisonous powder in drinking water supplies, Conradus Megenburgensis protested that this made no more sense than the other current theories, since plague occurred in places where there were no Jews. Seeing the logic of that, Pope Clement eventually issued a bull protecting the Jews after many had been burned alive and otherwise murdered without trial, starting at Narbonne and Carcassone in the normally tolerant south of France and spreading far and wide to reach Strasburg in the northeast, where at least 2,000 were lynched in February 1349 before the plague even arrived. And on the blood lust went, travelling through Germany and the Baltic countries. Where a trial did take place, there was no problem getting confessions by the use of sustained torture.[4] The plague eventually made it across the North Sea to Scandinavia in May 1349 when an English ship with a cargo of wool drifted ashore near Bergen, every man aboard having died at sea. Curious locals going on board carried the plague ashore with them to strike high and low. Even Sweden's King Magnus II lost his brothers Haakon and Cnut in the following year.[5]

Living at Avignon's papal court at the same time as Raimundus was a physician named Gui de Chauliac. Observing that buboes were not always present in plague victims affected by an even more violent and lethal form of the disease, he wrote:

> The mortality lasted seven months. It was of two types.
> The first lasted two months, with continuous fever and
> coughing of blood. Men suffer in their lungs and breathing
> and whoever have these corrupted, or even slightly attacked,
> cannot live beyond two days. The second form lasted for
> the rest of the period, also with continuous fever, but with
> [buboes] on the external parts, principally on the armpits
> and groin. From this one died in five days.[6]

A later chronicler describe in horrific detail how the Black Death deprived its victims of pity and sympathy because the symptoms were so disgusting that the sick became objects more of detestation and horror than of pity: 'All the matter which exuded from their bodies let off an unbearable stench: sweat, excrement, spittle, breath so fetid as to be overpowering; urine turbid, thick, black or red.'[7]

When plague reached Spain, it may have been a different disease – possibly typhus – because Ibn Khatimah recorded only seventy or so deaths daily at the peak of the infection. He argued that the stench might permanently pollute the air, so that in the centre of a formerly infected area no flame could afterwards burn, nor human breathe; on the periphery, he believed, was a zone of partial corruption where there was still a risk of death. It was recommended to burn fragrant wood, juniper and rosemary being among the favourites; a few tried throwing on the fire a mixture of sulphur, arsenic and antimony.[8] Since sulphur fumes destroy bacteria, this may have worked.[9] More desperate inhalation counsel included a recommendation to spend long periods with one's head over a stinking latrine or cesspool, to counteract a different kind of foul air, but many people fell in and drowned.

Khatimah's contemporary, also in Moorish Spain, Ibn al Khatib (1313–1375) did not disagree, but argued that the pollution of the air was only temporary. Another Arab living at Salé in Italy with a good supply of food named Ibn abu Madyan walled his entire household up inside his house. Emerging when the plague had died down, they all survived, giving the lie to the theory of polluted air.

Foreshadowing the travel restrictions imposed during the 2020 virus pandemic, the town council of Pistoia issued a proclamation nine pages long on 2 May 1348 forbidding travel to the regions of Pisa or Lucca; nor could anyone already there return home. Street markets were closely supervised, especially to prevent discarded waste food feeding rats. Funerals could be attended only by relatives of the deceased.[10] Foreshadowing the confusion of the British government in 2020, the municipal council of Orvieto did nothing to prepare for the plague when it was obviously drawing nearer, thus condemning its citizens to four months of hell from what appears to have been septicaemic plague, with 500 victims a day dying within twenty-four hours of infection. The city's lasting memorial to the plague, still standing, is its truncated cathedral; after work stopped due to the infection, the funds set aside were diverted to more urgent matters and building was never resumed.[11]

From Montpellier, the plague raced inland into a nation, a large part of which was riven by war between England's King Edward III and Philippe IV de Valois over the claim of Edward to Gascony, the rump of the once vast Plantagenet possessions in France. This was, to use a modern term, total war, with each side burning crops, cutting down fruit trees and uprooting vines on each foray into enemy territory. They also destroyed agricultural machinery in defiance of the Church's ban, preventing the peasants from recovering wasted land. As the armies traversed the ruined landscape, plague travelled with them, to infect the starving peasants.

By 1350 it seemed that the worst was over in France, but next door in southern Germany it began its depredations in June 1348 and crept from there up the valley of the Moselle and into North Germany, reaching Frankfurt-am-Main in the summer of 1349 and there killing 2,000 people in the space of two months. In Mainz 6,000 died; in Munster 11,000; in Erfurt 12,000.[12] To deflect the wrath of God a movement calling itself the Brethren of the Cross sprang up, its members practising self-flagellation to the point of drawing blood three times a day. There was an element of exhibitionism as the bands of Flagellants, several thousand strong approached a town weeping and singing. People turned out to witness the spectacle at every stop. Some locals joined in, as though going on crusade, but the sheer numbers of participants demanding, sometimes with menaces, both shelter and food at each stop strained the resources of monasteries and even municipalities.

Although to begin with the movement stayed within reasonable bounds, by the middle of 1349, the various bands were out of control, attacking anyone who remonstrated with them and especially Jews and lepers, both of which categories died from the plague as did other men. In a reverse of the twentieth century Holocaust, Poland was a haven of safety, possibly because King Kazimierz III Wielki, known in English as Casimir the Great, listened to the advice of his Jewish mistress, Esterka. In Spain, Portuguese pilgrims were attacked; in Aragon English ones too. Magistrates, bishops and archbishops banned them from entering cities. Pope Clement had himself encouraged some mortification of the flesh as public penance in Avignon, but in October 1349 he published a bull denouncing the Brethren's contempt of the Church. A few Flagellants crossed the Channel to England, but were swiftly deported back to Flanders.

Along the Mediterranean littoral, plague hopped from port to port, reaching Spain, where it lasted until 1420; arriving late in Russia, it lasted there until 1400; and in Germany it was present somewhere in the country 1485–1627.

Between 1348, when it first arrived in London and the Great Plague in 1666 there was a major epidemic of the plague in the capital roughly every two or three decades, killing between a 1/5 and 1/4 of the city's population each time. The 1348 plague began in England in the autumn and reached Wales in March 1349, both by sea through the west coast ports and by land from Herefordshire, Shropshire and Cheshire. It struck fiercely into the native Welsh-speaking population living in the hills, whose diet was lacking in nutrition, but also affected the better-fed English settlers who had established a manorial system in the valleys, producing a kind of anarchy as the surviving hill-dwellers came down by night to steal the property of the dead colonisers. The Welsh robbers were not so much expecting to find valuables as pots and pans, oddments of food and animals that could be driven off. Playing on the common Welsh man's name Dafydd, this was the origin of the nursery rhyme that endured into the twentieth century: 'Taffy was a Welshman. Taffy was a thief. / Taffy came to our house and stole a leg of beef.' Some historians even think that the anarchy which began during the plague played a large part in the later rebellion of the last Welsh prince of Wales Owain Glyndŵr (1359–1416?), who fought against English hegemony beginning in 1400.

Even less is known of the plague in Ireland, also partly colonised by English settlers. Most probably arriving through Irish Sea trade, principally with Bristol, the disease rampaged inland. The Franciscan annalist John Clyn (1286–1349) at St Francis' Abbey in Kilkenny recorded its arrival on Irish soil:

> In the months of September and October [1348, people] came in great numbers from every part of Ireland to the pilgrimage centre of that Molyngis. So great were their numbers that on many days it was possible to see thousands of people flocking there: some through devotion but the majority indeed through fear of the plague. It began in Dublin at Howth and Drogheda [which] were almost entirely destroyed and emptied of inhabitants, so that in Dublin alone, between the beginning of August and Christmas, 14,000 people died.[13]

Elsewhere, he wrote, the plague

virtually depopulated villages and cities, and castles and towns. It was so contagious that whosoever touched the sick or the dead was immediately infected and died; and the penitent and the confessor were carried together to the grave. Through fear and dread men scarcely dared to perform the offices of piety and pity in visiting the sick and burying the dead. Many died of boils and abscesses, and pustules on their shins or under the armpits; others died frantic with the pain in their head, and others spitting up blood. By Christmas of 1348 twenty-five friars had died in the Franciscan Convent of Drogheda, and twenty-three in the Convent of the same Order in Dublin. In Kilkenny, from Christmas Day to the 6th day in March, eight Friars Preachers died of it. Scarcely ever did just one person die in a house. Commonly husband, wife, children, and servants went [together along] the way of death.

And I, Brother John Clyn, of the Order of Friars Minors, wrote in this book those notable things, which happened in my time, which I saw with my own eyes, or which I learned from persons worthy of credit. And lest things worthy of remembrance should perish with time, and fall away from the memory of those who are to come after us, I, seeing these many evils, and the whole world lying as it were among the dead, waiting for death til (sic) it come, as I have truly heard and examined, so have I reduced these things to writing. And lest the writing should perish with the writer, and the work fail together with the workman, I leave parchment for continuing the work, if haply any man survive, and any race of Adam escape this pestilence and continue the work which I have commenced.[14]

After 'waiting for death til it come', Brother John's work ceased abruptly on 17 June 1349 when, it seems, the plague claimed also his life. Before then, after the year-long siege of Calais, King Edward III was forced to halt his war in France by the plague killing his soldiers and citizens alike.

For whatever reasons, little detailed history of the plague in Scotland is available. It touched parts of southern Scotland in the autumn of 1349, but caused few deaths until the following spring. Some historians ascribe this delay to the reluctance of rats to find new quarters in cold weather. A clerk in holy orders who may have been the almoner of Aberdeen cathedral was the chronicler John of Fordoun (died 1384). His major work was the *Chronica Gentis Scotorum,* which includes the following:

> In the Year 1350 there was in the kingdom of Scotland so great a pestilence and plague among men as from the beginning of the world had never been heard of by man [killing] nearly a third of mankind. This evil led to a strange kind of death. The flesh of the sick was somehow puffed out and swollen and they [survived] for barely two days. Men shrank from it so much that, through fear of contagion, sons, fleeing as from the face of leprosy or an adder, durst not go and see their parents in the throes of death.[15]

Not much to go on, but contemporaries of John of Fordoun reiterated that about a third of the population died – a lower proportion that was generally quoted in Europe. Possibly, this was due to many Scottish people still living in places remote from the contagion of towns.

South of the border, in England during the first eighteen months of this plague it killed almost half of London's population, estimated at 70,000 or more if the villages outside the city wall are counted. At the peak of the outbreak, it was impossible to bury all the corpses in individual graves, so huge plague pits were dug and the bodies tipped in several deep. The bodies of children were thrown in between the adult dead, to save space. Occasionally a person not actually dead recovered consciousness in them and had to fight his or her way through the bodies lying on top, presumably later dying from contagion. A number of these pits have been excavated, permitting full genome testing of teeth and especially the calculus deposited on unbrushed teeth to confirm that bubonic plague was the cause of death, although there is, at the time of writing, a revisionist theory that this was not the cause, or not the sole cause, of this epidemic. Zoologist Dr Graham Twigg published in 1984 a book entitled *The Black Death: A Biological Reappraisal* which contains his argument for the pandemic not being due to bubonic plague. Some other scientists agree with him; others do not.

Whichever theory is right, the social consequences of all the deaths were important. Fields were unploughed or not sown. Even such crops as did ripen often rotted in the fields because of the shortage of agricultural labourers to harvest them. Except for the very rich, food was in short supply, even for the reduced numbers in the towns. That this changed in a matter of months was due not to Edward III and his court, but to surviving peasants in pockets untouched by the plague moving into houses that had belonged to dead victims and taking over the land they had farmed.

Although there were no means of collating figures of deaths internationally at the time, it has been estimated that more than half the population of Europe died in this pandemic. What terrified people was not just the horrible sight of the black buboes on the skin of many victims, the high fevers and intolerable pain, but also the rapidity of death, sometimes just hours after infection and rarely more than a few days later. In 1518 the first comprehensive measures to contain the plague included hanging a sheaf of straw outside plague-ridden houses for the quarantine period of forty days, to warn off potential visitors. If any person from such a house did go outside, it was obligatory to carry a white stick, to discourage any close personal contact. Later, a red or black cross was painted on the doors of houses where plague victims were locked in, often accompanied with the legend 'God have mercy on us.' The corpses were carted away in the night, the men handling them smoking tobacco in pipes as a supposed prophylactic against the infection of the bodies they were handling.[16] The weed had only arrived in Europe a century before and was credited with magical properties.

In a city like London, black rats, which are excellent climbers, often made their nests in the thatch roofs. Since there were usually no ceilings below the roofs, a flea falling from the thatch could easily find itself a new, human host below. Although the landward boundaries of the city were protected by the original Roman walls to keep human enemies at bay, that proved no barrier for the rats.

After every pandemic commerce and industry have suffered. Because the medieval epidemics killed mostly the working poor, in city and country alike, there was a shortage of labourers afterwards. In the countryside most of the peasantry had been serfs, tied to the land where they had been born. Now survivors demanded wages and, if this was refused, slipped away in search of better pickings. That left the landowner having to pay new workers, which increased his cost of production of the saleable surplus in a society badly affected financially by all the deaths. An alternative was to divide the property and rent it out as smallholdings for cash. The gravity of the labour shortage caused the enactment of the Ordinance of Labourers in 1349 and the Statute of Labourers in 1351.[17] But the damage was done and led eventually to the Peasants' Revolt led by Wat Tyler, lasting from May to November 1381. If the spark that ignited this uprising was the poll tax imposed by the ill-advised 14-year-old Richard II to finance his French war, the massing of tens of thousands of protesters marching on London from south and north had its beginnings in the changes wrought on English society by the plague. Despite being known as a revolt of peasants, many other people joined in.

The citizens of London understood this when they opened the gates to them and let them attack the Tower, foreshadowing the later storming of the Bastille. Revisionists may argue otherwise, but the rejection of feudalism and serfdom that followed the first Black Death and the replacement of barter by the use of money as a means of exchange of goods and services was an important stage in the evolution of a modern society with free movement of labour. Religion was still important, but the Church had been shown sadly wanting. How many people in Britain at the time had even heard of the Greek philosopher Epicurus or read his test of divinity?

> If God is willing to prevent evil, but not able to do so,
> he is not omnipotent.
> If he is able, but not willing,
> Then he is malevolent.
> If he is both able and willing,
> Whence cometh evil?
> If he is neither able nor willing,
> Why call him god?

But one did not need to be a philosopher to know that the foundations of the feudal era were crumbling and outbreaks of plague played their part in this. In 1563, with Queen Elizabeth I on the throne, 7,000 English troops commanded by Lord Warwick occupied the French port of Le Havre. On 27 June, Warwick wrote home that his soldiers were dying from disease at the rate of sixty a day. Two days later, the total so far reached 500, and by the end of June, less than half of Warwick's men were fit for combat. On 29 July he received Elizabeth's permission to yield the port-city to the besieging army of the French king Charles X. Although the queen ordered the soldiery returning from Le Havre to be welcomed back with honour, they brought with them this new disease. The symptoms were different from those of previous plagues, and seem to have been confined to violent fever with high temperatures alternating with chills, parched mouth, irritating rashes on chest and loins, crippling headaches and terrible fatigue ending in death. Whatever this new plague was, it spread fast, killing a third of the population of Lyons in the east of France that year and reaching the Mediterranean coastal cities by the following summer. Then, a harsh winter seemed to kill off the pathogen – for a while.

On both sides of the Channel the outbreaks of disease caused peasant revolts and people of all strata of society came to doubt, not just whether there was a god, but what was the use of a monarch who could not impose stability. It was all very well for James I (king of England, r. 1603–1625) to proclaim the divine right of kings, but his reign commenced with a plague outbreak, described by John Davies, a Hereford schoolmaster thus:

> Cast out your dead, the carcass-carrier cries,
> Which he by heaps in [unconsecrated] graves inters ...
> The London lanes, themselves thereby to save,
> Did vomit out their undigested dead,
> Who by cartloads are carried to the grave.[18]

Death sought all classes, although those with the money to escape the towns for a second home in the country – the further away, the better – had the best chance. These plague refugees were not just the nobility, but included lawyers, merchants, judges and doctors, whose abandoned city homes were broken into by poorer people with nothing to lose, as they saw it. Such was the desolation described by the poet Abraham Holland (1596–1626), himself to die of the plague:

A noon in Fleet Street now can hardly show
That press which midnight could, not long ago.
Walk through the woeful streets (whoever dare
Still venture on the sad infected air).
So many marked houses you shall meet
As if the city were one Red Cross Street.[19]

Another poet, John Taylor, who was bargeman to James I's queen, Anne of Denmark, wrote of the 1625 plague:

In some whole street, perhaps, a shop or twain
Stands open for small takings and less gain.
And every closed window, door and stall
Makes every day seem a solemn festival.
All trades are dead, or almost out of breath
But such as live by sickness and by death.
… my multitude of graves that gaping wide
Are hourly fed by carcases of men.
Those hardly swallowed, they be fed again.
… Dead coarses [sic] carried and recarried still
While fifty corpses scarce one grave doth fill.[20]

The time was not far off when a ruling English king's divine right would be terminated by the executioner's axe. At the time of writing in late 2020, one wonders what cataclysmic social and economic consequences the Covid-19 pandemic will produce in the coming years.

Chapter 5

A Plethora of Plagues

The practice of bleeding the sick, whether or not guided by any theory of emunctories, and the application of medieval medicine containing snake venom, dried and crushed organs and excrement of animals and various herbs, was useless against disease. Some doctors trying their best and actually visiting the sick in time of plague were recognisable by the distinctive beaked headgear in their protective clothing. The beak was functional, containing aromatic herbs to combat the foul stench of sickness and decomposition. Some patients recovered. Otherwise, infected households were locked in and abandoned to divine mercy, the bodies thrown into mass graves after death. Modern research that casts doubt on the importance of the rat-flea vector, blaming instead human fleas and lice in transferring the pathogen directly from one person to another, indicates that instinctively fleeing to the country was an excellent idea.[1] Those affluent enough left the crowded towns, but the poorer city-dwellers had nowhere else to go.

Some Christians blamed this plague on Jews to justify pogroms. In January 1349 the Swiss town of Basel burned alive all its Jewish inhabitants. In Speyer, Jews were tortured and burned at the stake; many shut themselves up in their houses, which were then burned down with them inside. As a measure of what was seen as preventive hygiene, the burned corpses were placed in wine casks, which were then set adrift on the Rhine, to infect towns down-river. In February the city authorities of Strasbourg marched all the inhabitants of Jewish ethnicity to a local cemetery and burned them at the stake there. In Worms, the Jewish community, threatened with death at Christian hands, locked themselves in their homes and set fire to them, choosing to perish by their own hands.[2] In southern France, where Occitan-speaking population was less rigidly monotheist, they had a word *concivença* which means universal tolerance. There, the Jews were safe, many seeking and finding a haven after fleeing to the region of

Aquitaine and the Mediterranean counties. Yet across the Pyrenees in Spain and Catalunya Christians vented their anti-Semitism in pogroms. More northern cities targeted beggars, pilgrims, lepers and nomads of all descriptions. Among those who took pleasure in killing Jews were many Flagellants, or Brethren of the Cross.

Before seeming to die out by herd immunity, this episode of the Black Death had killed over 50 million victims, or nearly half the population of Europe. Yet it continued to lurk in pockets, awaiting ideal conditions to re-emerge. Workers excavating the tunnels for London's new Crossrail train line in 2013 discovered some skeletons buried in the Clerkenwell area of London on the site of a medieval monastery outside the medieval city walls. Tests revealed the presence of *Y. pestis*, also that while some victims died in the original epidemic of 1348–53 and were buried tidily, others from later outbreaks in 1361, 1368–69, 1371, 1375, 1390, 1405 and in the 1430s showed signs of injury before their corpses were hurled into the pit, hinting at a period of lawlessness.

The Franciscan friar Michele of Piazza described the symptoms when the disease first arrived in Sicily:

> Then a boil developed on the thighs, or on their upper arms a boil ... This infected the whole body, so that the patient violently vomited blood. This vomiting of blood continued without intermission for three days, there being no means of curing it, and then the patient died. Soon men hated each other so much that, if a son was attacked by the disease, his father would not care for him. If, in spite of all, he dared approach him, he was immediately infected and ... was bound to expire within three days ... all those dwelling in the same house, even the cats and other domestic animals, followed him to the grave. Soon the corpses were lying forsaken in the houses. No ecclesiastic, no son, no father and no relation dared to enter.[3]

The Franciscan monk also noted the arrival in Sicilian ports of twelve Genoese galleys coming from the Crimea. Yet, according to him, while the crews seemed perfectly healthy 'anyone who only spoke to them was seized by a mortal illness and in no way could avoid death. The infection spread to everyone who had any intercourse with the diseased.

Those infected felt themselves penetrated by a pain throughout their whole bodies.'[4] Forced to put to sea, the galleys continued to Genoa. Although the crews seemed perfectly healthy, within a few days, the plague was rife. When the plague reached Florence, Giovanni Boccaccio described the symptoms similarly, adding: 'The victims' thirst was unquenchable and some of them ran naked through the streets, screaming, and plunged into water cisterns. Others went completely mad with the pain and even threw themselves out of windows. Death was truly a merciful release.'[5]

The notary Gabriele de' Mussi recorded:

> The cemeteries failing, it was necessary to dig trenches to bury the corpses. Whole families were frequently thrown together in the same pit. One Oberto de Sasso, who had come from an infected place to the Church of the Friars Minor to make his will, summoned a notary, witnesses and neighbours. All these, together with sixty others, died within a short space of time.[6]

The Italian humanist poet Petrarch died suddenly on 19 July 1374, probably from the plague. He wrote to his brother, the only monk who survived from the community of thirty-five in his monastery:

> Sorrow is on all sides. I wish, my brother, that I had never been born, or at least had died before these times. Will posterity ever believe these things, when we who see them, can scarcely credit them? We would think we were dreaming if we did not see the city in mourning with funerals, and on returning home, find it empty and thus know that what we lament is real.[7]

From Italy, the plague travelled into France, where the exiled Pope Clement VI came up with an original idea to rid the city of Avignon of the many corpses lying in the streets after all the cemeteries were full. He declared the River Rhône to be 'consecrated ground' so that the dead could be thrown into it in a semblance of Christian burial.[8]

The orthodox Christians of Cyprus feared that those who survived the plague would be outnumbered by their Muslim servants, who would take control of the island. Their remedy was to murder all the servants in a long afternoon of massacre.

By December 1348 the plague had crossed the English Channel, and was to return to London forty times in 300 years, eventually killing up to 5 million people in England. Because the bacillus was transmitted by fleas on cats and dogs in addition to rats, preventive measures included a wholesale massacre of thousands of pets. Some 40,000 dogs and 200,000 cats were slaughtered. There was a sort of prophylactic logic in the slaughter, but, left alive, those dogs and cats might have killed many rodents.

An interesting survey conducted under the aegis of the London School of Economics traces the development of London during the century of repeated plagues beginning in 1560.[9] After analysing records of nearly a million deaths and over a half-million births, the conclusion was that the plagues of 1563, 1593, 1603, 1625 and 1665-6 had similar effects, with a spike in the autumn raising deaths to nearly six times the normal level. Each time, about a fifth of London's population died in the space of a few months. An exception is the plague of 1636 when, for reasons unknown, deaths were only 2.3 per cent up on the norm for non-plague years. Perhaps the records for that year are incomplete?

If isolation was the only protection, one might think that Iceland would be safe. Yet it suffered two plagues in the fifteenth century. The problem was that the island imported many goods that could not be produced locally – like timber, grain, sugar – from Norway and Scotland. A document called *The New Annal* records the arrival of plague in September 1402 in a ship that reached the port of Hvalfjördur. It travelled from there on land for 200 miles in sixteen weeks, undeterred by the onset of winter and the virtual absence of towns, most Icelanders then living in remote farmsteads. *The New Annal* calls the following year 'the year of great mortality', with an estimated 60 or 70 per cent of Icelanders dying. Before the end of the century, the development of London gave rise to the century of repeated plagues beginning in 1560–65. When the plague returned, an Icelander named Jón Egilsson gave a sad picture of this visit: 'In this plague the mortality was so great that no one remembered or had heard of anything like it. On most farms, only two or three people survived, sometimes [infants] sucking on their dead mothers. At Tungufell's-Manga, where there had been nine children, [only] two or three were left alive.'[10] Not surprisingly, given the rigours of life in Iceland, it was to take 500 years for population figures to return to the original level.

A thousand miles to the south, England was still suffering intermittently. The philosopher Erasmus of Rotterdam (1469–1536) wrote in 1514 that he deemed London unsafe to stay in, and commented that King Henry VIII (1491–1547) never walked in the city, but rode on horseback, to avoid close contact with the crowds.[11] King Henry was still on the throne in 1538 when plague struck York, then Durham and Newcastle upon Tyne. The eventual sign of plague – known as 'a Rede Cross sat uppon the dower [door]' – was first used during the outbreak at York in 1551. England's short-lived Protestant king Edward VI – son of Queen Jane Seymour and the only legitimate male heir of Henry VIII – was crowned at the age of 9 in 1547 and died six years later from what was termed 'an abcess on the lungs, having coughed up sputum often the colour of blood', which sounds like tuberculosis.

Susan Scott is a social historian who was consulting parish registers in the Record Office in Carlisle, where she came across this entry: 'A sore plague in Richmond, Kendal, Penreth, Carliel, Apulbie and othier places in Westmorland and Cumberland in the yere of oure Lord God 1598.'[12]

This entry from the time when Queen Elizabeth I was on the throne led her to:

Penrith Burial Registers 1597
September 22
Andrew Hogson, a stranger

HERE BEGONNE THE PLAGE (GOD PUNISMET) IN PENRITH

Those that are noted with thys letter P dyed of the infirmity and those that are noted with F are buried out on the fell.[13]

The visit of this outsider to Penrith, a small and fairly isolated market town of northwest England, nearly 300 miles from London, and where people had thought themselves out of reach of the plague, caused a terrible wave of mortality that lasted fifteen months, with every death recorded in the parish register. Ms Scott also discovered a brass plaque in the church recording the deaths in the Eden Valley:

PENRITH	2,260
KENDAL	2,500
RICHMOND	2,200
CARLISLE	1,196

Here lies a mystery, because Ms Scott knew that the inhabitants of Penrith only numbered 1,350 before the epidemic. Ignoring the plaque, she counted all the burials marked F in the parish register. They numbered about 640, which was bad enough, being half the population.

Whereas the early London plagues killed indiscriminately throughout the city, by 1665 the concentration of affluent families in the parishes within the Roman walls retarded mortality there to some extent, so that most plague deaths occurred in the poorer parishes outside the walls. This reflected the child mortality normal at the time. In the richer parishes a new-born had one chance in two of surviving into childhood; in poorer ones, it was only one chance in three. Outside the walls, the increasing number of suburban parishes had a mortality of 3.5 times normal in the early plague outbreaks, the poor northern suburbs of St Giles Cripplegate and Shoreditch always being among the worst hit. Yet, in 1665 the deaths in these parishes leaped up to six times the norm.

Why the difference? Historians investigating the 1613 plague in the Saxon town of Freiburg concluded that the lower mortality in the richer quarters was due to the greater protection against rats and their fleas afforded by the rich building their houses in masonry, whereas cheaper housing in the poorer quarters had timber frames with wattle-and-daub infill, easy for rodent parasites to penetrate. The first Stuart king of England James I (r. 1603–1625), reputedly had a nifty slogan defining the use of masonry as choosing 'bricks, not sticks' for home-building. The wattle-and-daub was quite fire-resistant when new, but old infill with flaking plasterwork left exposed patches of wattle that easily caught fire.

Complicating any mathematical analysis of mortality, it is not possible to define London as a single statistical entity. In the seventeenth century, population of the wealthier central parishes usually increased in plague-free years while the poorer parishes *normally* lost 10 per cent of population per annum by deaths, the deficit usually being made up by births and immigration from the provinces.

In 1563 London suffered the worst episode of plague in the sixteenth century with at least 20,136 inhabitants dying during this outbreak, mainly in the crowded poorer parishes and suburbs, where conditions were least sanitary. In this, the fifth year of the reign of Queen Elizabeth I most people seem to have forgotten the last plague a dozen or more years earlier and there was little control of the population. Then plague suddenly erupted in Derby, Leicester and London, spreading even to the English garrison at Le Havre under Lord Warwick, so reducing their numbers that Warwick had to surrender the town to the French besiegers. According to contemporary antiquarian and historian John Stow (c. 1525–1605), the first seventeen cases in London were recorded in Bills of Mortality for the week ending 12 June. While widely respected for his honesty, Stow was twice harassed by the Church because he had 'too many books' to be a loyal Protestant and was thus accused of papistry. This was at the time an alibi for maligning any man who uttered embarrassing truths.

The Virgin Queen charged churchwardens and curates to refuse entry to church to all caring for the sick, continuing after the deaths of the sick person(s) for several weeks. In Stratford-on-Avon people suffered seven distinct outbreaks of plague. On 11 July 1564 the parish registers again bore the entry *hic incepit pestis* – 'here began the plague'. By the following January, deaths totalled 220. Yet, an infant 9 months old, christened William, the son of John Shakespeare, a glover and sometime mayor of the town, survived and grew up to become England's major playwright.[14] This time, blue crosses were painted on the doors of infected houses and all stray animals killed 'for the avoidance of plague', their fleas presumably dying with them. In addition, the credence still given to the theory of plague-bearing miasmas caused the Queen's council to ordain that householders must light bonfires in the streets each evening at 7 p.m. to purify the air. Notwithstanding this, the weekly total of deaths climbed from 131 in the week ending 3 July to several hundred each week by the end of the month. The physician William Bullein recorded those 'fleeing the city in wagons, cartes and horses full loden with young barnes [children] for fear of the black Pestilence'.

The worst affected areas were in Turnagain Lane and Seacoal Lane, and in the parish of St Poulkar (St Sepulchre's church), where discarded fruit and vegetables from the weekday market made a rats' paradise. Attempts at cleaning up the streets were made by beadles employing rakers, who literally moved the stinking excrement and putrefaction with rakes, depositing it into open sewers or watercourses, where in dry weather, it stayed until sufficient rain fell to move it onward. Some of these men drowned in over-full cesspools. In 1357 Edward III complained to the lord mayor that his pleasure in travelling down the Thames was marred by the stench from the 'dung, lay-stalls and other filth dumped on the banks'. Lay-stalls were pens for cattle brought to market, also used for dumping dung. The several tributaries of the London Thames acted as open sewers. The Fleet river had many privies built out over it, all the solid waste from which choked it frequently, so that no water could flow.

Among the people infected were doctors, one of whom contracted the plague when staying with a friend who did not at first present any symptoms. The doctor survived; his friend did not. Realising that affluence and rank were no safeguard, Queen Elizabeth I commanded the governor of the Tower to remove Lady Katherine Grey – sister of the executed 'nine-days queen' Lady Jane – and Katherine's husband the earl of Hertford, for fear that the plague might infect the insanitary ancient prison. Their crime was having married without the queen's permission. The court decamped from London to Windsor where, outside the walls a gallows was erected, on which to hang anyone coming from London and possibly carrying the infection. Likewise, potentially dangerous merchandise from London was refused entry into Windsor. In September the weekly death toll in the capital abandoned by the royal family surged past 1,000, to reach 1,828 in the first week of October.

The plague seems to have started in the pneumonic form, changing to the bubonic as the summer warmed up. Nearly two years were to pass before the last Londoners died. It was ordained that all infected houses should have their doors and windows boarded up, with a forty-day quarantine imposed on any survivors. Later the Common Council decreed that no house that had been infected could be rented out, in case infection lingered. This was quite possible, since fleas can survive a long time without feeding, and would attack any newcomer months after their last blood meal. With the cooler autumn weather, the plague seemed to lose its momentum; deaths declined to less than twenty a week after Christmas and, by the end of January, the city was considered plague-free.

How far one can rely on the weekly Bills of Mortality compiled for each parish, is uncertain. Today's medical practitioners easily distinguish between plague and typhus but Charles Murchison, the eminent Victorian specialist at the London Fever Hospital and St Thomas's Hospital noted that some symptoms of plague and typhus were almost identical, except for the buboes on the lymphatic glands. Yet typhus can also produce swollen lymph glands and quasi-buboes. Less experienced doctors could also easily confuse the petechial spots caused by bleeding in the skin of typhus victims and the famous *ring o'roses* known as 'God's tokens' on the skin of plague sufferers. Like plague, typhus can quickly produce an agonising death. Plague kills both adults and children; typhus rarely kills the young. But there were also rampant outbreaks of smallpox, dysentery and influenza. The last-named killer owns an Italian name *influenza* (influence in English), the original idea being that it was caused by the influence of the stars. Syphilis, dubbed in English 'the French pox' with the French calling it *la maladie de Naples* and the Italians *la malattia francesa* was, like gonorrhoea, always in wait for the unwary – and other occasional killers like anthrax were always waiting for their moments to strike.

The city of Milan financed a public health authority since the 1400s, which systematically monitored plague cases on its northern frontier, concentrating on principal trade routes, including those roads leading toward the various Alpine passes. But this collapsed during the Italian Wars of 1499–1559, which caused recurring food shortages, plagues, and pestilences over all northern Italy. Foreign troops repeatedly crossed the mountains into northern Italy, often bringing plague with them.

In 1629 troops returning from the Thirty Years' War carried plague to Mantua. Over the next two years, it progressed to Verona, Milan, Florence and Venice, whence it spread to kill another 280,000 people in Italian cities. In Milan and Venice, the authorities confined victims in isolated plague houses and burned all their possessions. In addition, the Venetians isolated victims on the islands in the lagoon, formerly used to confine lepers (they are still uninhabited), but nevertheless lost one-third of the city's population of 140,000. The social and economics consequences of epidemics and pandemics, including Covid-19 can never be predicted with confidence. Historians date the commercial and political decline of the former world power of the Venetian republic to the fatalities caused by this plague.

Before the advent of modern sanitation and health practices, there were so many plagues and epidemics that it is often difficult to identify them, even when described by contemporary writers. Until the last years of the twentieth century, it was believed by researchers and historians that all the plagues which beset medieval Europe were variants of bubonic plague. However zoologist Professor C. J. Duncan decided on the evidence of haemorrhagic fevers in the Nile Valley 1500–1350 BCE, a Mesopotamian diagnostic handbook c. 721–453 BCE, the plague of Athens 430 BCE, the plague of Justinian 541–42 CE, plagues in Islamic countries 627–744 CE, plague in Asia Minor and the Levant 1345–48, the European plagues of 1345–1679, Scandinavian plagues 1710–11 and sporadic plagues in Poland during the eighteenth century that the disease in all these cases was a viral haemorrhagic fever from Ethiopia with an incubation period of thirty-two days. [15]

This, he argued, was the reason why quarantine was changed in Italy from thirty to forty days. England stayed with this quarantine until the sixteenth century, and then reverted to thirty days. When this was found ineffective, England returned to a forty-day period. After 1550 the improvement in transport and the continued growth in the population of towns increased the speed of spread, the frequency and the ferocity of plagues. Measures such as forcing victims into pest houses and locking whole families into their houses were ineffective because the contagion was more rampant *before* symptoms showed. Professor Duncan quoted Daniel Defoe's book, written with the benefit of hindsight, mentioning

> apparently healthy people who harbour the disease but have not yet exhibited symptoms. Such a person was in fact a poisoner, a walking destroyer perhaps for a week or a fortnight before his death, who might have ruined those he would have hazarded his life to save … breathing death upon them, even perhaps his tender kissing and embracings of his own children.

Professor Duncan held that patients with bubonic plague were not normally infectious and could be nursed in open wards. The incubation period is typically only two to six days; the characteristic symptom is the bubo; a patient's temperature can rise as high as 39.4 degrees Centigrade (102.3 degrees Fahrenheit). Most patients die between the third and sixth day; if they are alive on the seventh day, they may survive. However, in about 5 per cent of cases *Y. pestis* reaches the lungs, the patient coughs out bacteria in the sputum and droplets may be inhaled by anyone nearby, infecting them with the pneumonic form and killing them rapidly if no treatment is available.

So, was it the Black Death, or some haemorrhagic fever? The jury is still out, as they say, and it is possible both plague and typhus coincided. On the Third Crusade (1189–92] both King Richard the Lionheart and the French monarch Philippe Auguste were among hundreds of victims in the European armies of arnaldia, or *leonardie* in French. This was an unpleasant, possibly viral contagious fever with copious and debilitating sweating and skin rashes, and which caused the nails, teeth and hair to fall out, lips to peel painfully and whole strips of skin to fall away from the body. Both monarchs survived, but Philippe's hair never grew back and he was so feeble after the attack that he had to return to Europe. Richard returned to the fray and pulled off some clever exercises in generalship, which all came to nothing in the end, leaving him to beg a single ship from the Templars, in which to make the return journey – which ended in the disaster of his imprisonment in Austria and Germany.[16]

The infection may have been carried back to Europe with the returning crusaders. Was it a modified form of arnaldia, or another disease that caused several medieval and later epidemics in England called the 'sweating syknes' (medical name *sudor anglicus*)? This was characterised by high fever and stinking sweats – although, given the rarity of bathing in those times, the stench have been the sufferer's body odour when the fever caused clothing to be torn off in desperation – as well as intolerable itching and unbearable headaches. Violent fits were followed by somnolence, respiratory difficulties, convulsions and heart and kidney problems. Victims died after twenty-four agonising hours.

But there may be no connection, for the *syknes* first became rampant in England after the Battle of Bosworth Field, when Henry Tudor killed Richard III on 22 August 1485, although at the time the disease was blamed on mercenaries bringing it from France.

This outbreak lasted until January 1486, but returned in 1507–08, 1517–18, 1528–29 and 1551, when it caused 1,000 deaths in London during one week – including two lord mayors and six aldermen – and in some towns carried off a third of the population, being no respecter of rank. Cardinal Wolsey fell victim more than once, and recovered. So many members of Henry VIII's court were infected that Bluff King Hal changed his residence frequently, leaving behind the sufferers in the hope of avoiding the infection. After that, it apparently died out as an epidemic, although individual cases continued to occur. In France, it was known as *la suette des Picards* – the Picardy Sweat – although this may have been a variant or a similar disease entirely. It last appeared in northern France in 1906.

In England, the outbreak of 1551 enabled a brilliant and very successful doctor to give his name to a Cambridge college. After years spent travelling abroad, Norwich-born Dr John Kays returned to England calling himself Dr Johannus Caius, Latin being the language of the medical profession. Observing in detail the symptoms, and charging his wealthy patients for the privilege of dying in his care, he wrote *An Account of the Sweating Sickness in England.*[17] Educated at Gonville Hall in Cambridge, by then fallen on hard times, he donated generously to his *alma mater*, which changed its name to Gonville and Caius College.

Speculation as to the cause of sweating sickness continued. When a similar malady manifested itself among the Navajo people living in New Mexico during 1993, researchers blamed it on the Sin Nombre virus. The Spanish name simply meaning 'nameless', this pathogen is classed as a hantavirus, causing HPS – hantavirus pulmonary syndrome. Hantaviruses are long-time enemies of humankind, often transmitted by the urine of infected rats in the waters of tropical streams. In New Mexico, the virus was in the urine and excrement of field mice, inhaled by people cleaning an infested barn, or even just brushing away rodents' droppings on the ground and, in the process, releasing into the air they were breathing minute particles of contaminated dust.

And what is one to make of the convulsive affliction known as St Vitus' Dance, choreomania, the dancing plague or Sydenham's chorea? St Vitus was a third-century Sicilian healer who cured Emperor Diocletian of 'his demons' by laying his hands on the emperor's head, and thus became associated with neurological problems. Little good did it do him: Diocletian had him martyred by being thrust into a cauldron of boiling water. First noted in the seventh century, the dancing mania then known as *le triste mal* recurred sporadically until the mid-seventeenth century, notably at Aachen in 1374. Sometimes, bystanders were violently attacked, if they refused to join in the dance. After the second plague, it reappeared and spread like a virus over the European continent, affecting hundreds of thousands of men, women and children, who would dance together for hours in the streets or open places, seemingly in a trance, until they collapsed, ecstatic, exhausted or, in some cases, dead on the spot. In Italy, it was known as *tarantismo* and ascribed to the bite of a tarantula spider. The sixteenth-century Swiss-German doctor and philosopher Paracelsus (1494–1541) – real name Theothrastus von Hohenheim – wrote a treatise about St Vitus' Dance, which continued to be an umbrella term for convulsive conditions.[18] Was it a physical affliction or simply mass hysteria?

Chapter 6

The Great Plague Arrives in England

Plague returned to Europe in 1661, when it surfaced in Turkey, but did not reach England until after the Restoration, in 1665–66 when King Charles II and others rich enough fled to their country houses, leaving the poorer classes in the city, where between 75,000 and 100,000 people died from a population of 460,000.[1] Worldwide, it is estimated that deaths in this pandemic totalled anywhere from 75 million to 200 million. Daniel Defoe wrote *A Journal of the Plague Year*, but he was a child when it happened and wrote his book later for publication in 1722, using notes made at the time and hindsight. Fortunately, that most famous of English diarists Samuel Pepys stayed in London and wrote copiously *during* the plague, recording his experiences each day before going to bed and, as was his custom, mixing topics to include the financial problems of the spendthrift King Charles II, perpetually over-spending his allowance by parliament to the detriment of his navy and army in this time of war with the Dutch and the French, plus endless gossip and details of his own sex life. What is curious is that, although surrounded by the plague and people dying of it, Pepys gives it relatively little prominence.

He lived in very interesting times, playing truant from St Paul's school, aged 15, in order to witness the decapitation on 30 January 1649 of King Charles I outside the Banqueting House on Whitehall, where the block on which the king had to lay his head for the executioner's axe was so humiliatingly low that he had almost to lie down on the scaffold. During the nineteen years under the Lord Protector Oliver Cromwell and his ineffectual son, Richard Cromwell, Pepys served as a clerk, firstly in the Exchequer and then the Admiralty. With a keen ear for politics, he began his diary on 1 January 1660.

In May of that year, he travelled as secretary to his cousin Edward Montagu (1625–1672), first earl of Sandwich, to Holland, bringing the executed king's sons back to England from their long exile. The political chaos in England after the death of Oliver Cromwell is illustrated by

Lord Sandwich retaining power after serving the parliamentarian government, as did Vice-Admiral Sir John Lawson (c. 1615–1665), commander of the fleet, who had even blockaded the Thames at Gravesend for some months to force the city of London to stay loyal to parliament. Many other important people changed allegiance after the death of the lord protector, and were welcomed into the service of King Charles II. How else could he govern the country? He did, however sentence to death those who had signed the warrant for the execution of his father King Charles I.

With his politically important cousin and the other great and good, Samuel Pepys attended the coronation of Charles II in Westminster abbey on St George's Day, 23 April 1661. Two days earlier, Pepys had seen Charles and his current mistress, the very beautiful Barbara Palmer, at the theatre, where the monarch known to his subjects as 'the merry king' displayed what Pepys called 'a good deal of familiarity' towards her.[2] She had already borne him a daughter conceived on the day of his return to London, and was to present him with four more children, but she was not present at the coronation. On 13 July, Pepys was appointed Clerk of the Acts to the Navy Board, a position so remunerative that he refused an offer of £1,000 to step down in favour of a competitor. On first introducing Pepys to the Navy, Lord Sandwich had promised this bright young assistant that they would rise together, and so it proved. Charles did marry the Portuguese princess Catarina de Bragança on 21 May 1662, but despite three pregnancies she proved unable to carry a child to full term, so he continued begetting a litter of acknowledged illegitimate sons and daughters with a series of mistresses. The queen was hardly unaware with Barbara Palmer being made one of her ladies-in-waiting, to keep her near the king. He lavished upon her costly presents, which were a significant reason why his 1661–62 income from parliament of £1.2 million fell £300,000 short of his expenditure.

Pepys' famous diary was mostly written in a form of shorthand called Shelton's Tachygraphy, and records of his dalliances with women double-encoded in a mishmash of French, Italian, Latin and Spanish words, to confuse anyone who managed to break the code. The practice of using shorthand for his journal was not peculiar to him, but shared with other men in public life, like Sir Isaac Newton and US President Thomas Jefferson, who likewise had reason to keep their thoughts private from the prying eyes of servants. On 19 October 1663, the plague figured in the diary:

> Sir W. Batten and I took coach, and to the Coffee-house in Cornhill; where much talk about the Turk's proceedings, and that the plague is got to Amsterdam, brought by a ship from Argier [Algiers] and it is also carried to Hambrough [on the Isle of Wight, where the English ships were lying].

Pepys was naturally much taken up with affairs of the fleet. The first Anglo-Dutch war had ended in 1654, but by 1664 it was becoming obvious that hostilities would break out again over which country had the right to trade where on the planet. On 16 June of that year, Pepys noted: 'The talk upon the Change is that [Dutch Grand Admiral Michiel] de Ruyter is dead, with fifty men of his own ship, of the plague, at Cales [Calais].' Like most gossip, this was not wholly true: fifty crewmen may have died, but their admiral outlived them and the third Anglo-Dutch war, to die at the battle of Agosta on 22 April 1676 after a French cannon-ball tore off his left leg.

The winter of 1664 was unusually hard, with severe frosts from November to March 1665 producing chest problems for many otherwise healthy people. Pepys, however, pursued his usual pastimes. One of many reasons for his secretiveness in the diary was his habit of taking pleasure with women other than his attractive Huguenot wife Elizabeth. Before the plague reached England and the concurrent Dutch war, this sequence of several days gave no hint of what lay ahead, starting on 6 December 1664:

> So by and by Mrs Lane come and plucks me by the cloak to speak to me, and I was fain to go to her shop, and pretending to buy some bands made her go home, and by and by followed her, and there did what I would with her, and so after many discourses and her intreating me to do something for her husband, which I promised to do, and buying a little band of her, took leave. She is great with child and says I must be godfather, but I do not intend it. Thence by coach to the Old Exchange, and there hear that the Dutch are fitting their ships out again [for war].[3]

On 17 December 1664:

> Mighty talk there is of this Comet that is seen a'nights,
> and the King and Queene did sit up last night to see it,
> and did so, it seems. And tonight I thought to have done
> so too, but it is cloudy and so no stars appear. But I will
> endeavour it.

Comets were thought to be foretellers of misfortune to come, but next
morning Pepys was back to his normal routine:

> (Lord's Day) To church, where, God forgive me! I spent
> most of my time in looking [on] my new [brunette] Morena
> at the other side of the church, an acquaintance of Pegg
> Pen's. So home to [midday] dinner and then to my chamber
> to read Ben Johnson's *Cataline*, a very excellent piece.

On 19 December:

> Not finding Bagwell's wife as I expected, I to the 'Change
> and there walked up and down and then home. And she
> being come, I bid her go and stay at Mooregate for me.
> And after dinner I to the place and, not finding her, I to the
> 'Change and there found her waiting for me and took her
> away and to an ale house, and there I made much of her, and
> endeavoured to caress her, but *elle ne voulait pas*, which
> did vex me. A little to my office and to bed. My mind, God
> forgive me, too much running upon what I can *ferais avec
> la femme de Bagwell demain*.

On 20 December:

> Up and walked to Deptford, where after doing something
> at the [navy arsenal and] yard I walked, without being
> observed, with Bagwell home to his house, and there was
> very kindly used, and the poor people did get a dinner
> for me in their fashion, of which I also eat very well.
> After dinner I found occasion of sending him abroad, and

then alone *avec elle je tentais a faire ce que je voudrais et contre sa force je le faisais biens que passe a mon contentement.*[4]

To obtain Pepys' favour for her husband, Mrs Bagwell was willing to pleasure his employer, but reluctant to do so in the conjugal home, perhaps fearing her husband's return during the act. Advised by his patron Lord Sandwich that the comet was still to be seen, on 24 December, Pepys wrote:

> This evening I being informed did look and saw the Comet which is now, whether worn away or no, I know not, but appears not with a tail, but only is larger and duller than any other star, and is come to rise betimes, and to make a great arch, and is gone quite to a new place in the heavens than it was before: but I hope in a clearer night something more will be seen.

Apparently not too much worried by the comet, and having no inkling of what was to come, although comets were often taken for harbingers of evil in the offing, Pepys felt in very good health and wondered whether that was due to his lucky hare's foot he carried everywhere or the supposedly prophylactic turpentine pill he swallowed each day. At the end of that year he was congratulating himself on being worth over £500 more than at the end of 1663, making a grand total of £1,349 – a small fortune at the time. Very much the man about town, on 2 January 1665 he wrote:

> Agreed with Mrs Martin, and to her lodgings which she has now taken to lie in, in Bow Street, pitiful poor things, yet she thinks them pretty, and so they are for her condition I believe good enough. Here I did *ce que je voudrais avec* her most freely and, it having cost me 2 shillings in wine and cake upon her, I away sick of her impudence.

Although Mrs Bagwell was married, the prefix Mrs did not necessarily imply marriage at the time, but merely denoted an adult woman. Plagues were frequently part of medieval and renaissance life, kept track of by weekly Bills of Mortality, totalling the records kept by each parish in the city since 1603. In the first week of January 1665 Pepys was pleased that they recorded an increase of only seventy deaths, making a total of 253 in this visitation so far. But the following Bill recorded a jump of eighty-nine fatalities. On 13 January, he wrote: 'If the plague continues among us another yeare, the Lord knows what will become of us.'

On 23 January 1665:

> Finding Mrs Bagwell waiting at the office after [midday] dinner, away she and I to a cabaret where she and I have eat before, and there I had her company *tout* and had *mon plaisir* of *elle*. But strange to see how woman, notwithstanding her greatest pretences of love *a son mari* and religion, may be *vaincue*.

On 25 January Pepys heard that the king of France had publicly declared war on England, and confided to the diary – for few knew the state of the navy better than he – 'God knows,' he said, 'how little fit we are for it.' He enjoyed greatly his access to the new king and his brother the Duke of York, who had both moved further away from London, to Hampton Court: 'And the King come to me of himself, and told me, "Mr Pepys," said he, "I do give you thanks for your good service all this year, and assure you I am very sensible of it."'

From time to time Pepys mentions other towns like Chatham, Colchester, Deptford, Deal and Greenwich, where the plague was carrying off increasing numbers of victims. After 4 March 1665 with England at war with both the Dutch and the French, he noted the presence in the London streets of many women but few men, who dared not go out for fear that the roaming press gangs would carry them off willy-nilly to serve in the navy as impressed men.

Pepys' first mention of the plague was when it reached Amsterdam. Whether it did arrive in London in a parcel of woollen goods from Holland, as rumoured, or whether this was a piece of anti-Dutch fake news, in unknown. Next, it was in English-occupied Calais. On 12 April 1665 a woman named Margaret Ponteus in the parish of St Paul Covent Garden reportedly had the unfortunate distinction of being the first person to die of this outbreak of plague in London. On 30 April 1665 Pepys was alive to the increasing danger: 'Great fears of the Sickenesse here in the City, it being said that two or three houses are already shut up [here]. God preserve us all.' Pepys continued to live his life normally until the beginning of June, when, for the first time, he saw with his own eyes houses 'shut up' – the term then used for quarantine – 'and marked with a red cross upon the doors, and "Lord have mercy upon us" writ there'.

On 12 May the Privy Council Committee issued Plague Orders, requiring a general clean-up of the city streets, the destruction of all stray animals found there, the closure of infected houses and the placing of guards to prevent the occupants coming out, the reopening of London's five pest houses, which could only accommodate 600 cases in all.[5] The idea of the pest houses was to spare the families of plague victims the experience of being shut up with the sufferer. The 1665 epidemic reached London by several routes: directly from the south coast ports; from the west after a plague ship moored in Bristol harbour, the disease then spreading cross-country via Gloucester, where apparently nine out of every ten people died;[5] and more directly by the Severn and Thames rivers. Pepys commented,

> To my great trouble, hear that the plague is come into the city. Walked home; being forced thereto by one of my watermen falling sick yesterday, and it was God's great mercy that I did not go by water with them yesterday, for he fell sick on Saturday, and it is to be feared of the plague.

The waterman died among some 100,000 other Londoners; areas particularly affected were Whitechapel, Southwark and Clerkenwell. Pepys became increasingly troubled by the outbreak after seeing corpses being collected in the streets for burial. A number of his acquaintances died, including his own physician. On 29 June the Royal Court of Justice decamped from Westminster, heading for Syon House, then Hampton Court, then Salisbury one step ahead of the plague, and finally settling in Oxford in September. The royal family did not return to the capital for seven months. Many others who had homes in less plague-affected areas, also chose to flee, among then the famous mathematician and natural philosopher Isaac Newton, friend of Pepys and the philosopher John Locke, who abandoned Cambridge when the university shut down.

By 8 June 1665, Pepys was warning his wife Elizabeth to change her habitual route to a friend's house in order to avoid a plague-stricken area of London, but understandably he seemed more focused on Britain's naval victory against the Dutch a few days earlier. Two days later, he got word of plague cases on the street where his friend Dr Burnett, lived. Within a week, he was making arrangements for his wife, Elizabeth, to stay with friends outside of town until the end of the plague. Meanwhile, 112 people had died in London in the week since Pepys got the news about the naval victory. Around the same time, he started to mention friends and colleagues fleeing to the countryside, hoping to get away from the crowded city where the plague spread much faster.

When many people of his class left the plague-ridden capital to stay with family or in their second homes in the provinces, they were not greeted with open arms due to the fear of the locals that they had brought the plague with them. Pepys remained in London as an essential civil servant until ordered to relocate to an office at Greenwich. Even then, he commuted by river from there to his house in Seething Lane near the Tower of London, nervous that it might be burgled at night if he was not present to guard his illicit gains. On 24 May 1665 he wrote in his diary of a visit to a favourite coffee house, where gossip was more confusing than informative: 'All the news is of the Dutch [fleet putting to sea] and of the plague growing upon us in this towne, and of remedies against it, some saying one thing and some another.' In early June he remarked on the failure of the first preventive measures, strikingly similar to the first ineffectual measures when Covid-19 attacked England in early 2020. On 7 June, he wrote: 'I did in Drury Lane see two or three houses marked with a red cross on the doors and "Lord have mercy on us" writ there – which was a sad sight for me.'

Sad sights abounded on all sides. Ten days later, on 17 June Pepys recorded an unpleasant incident:

> It struck me very deep this afternoon going with a hackney coach from my Lord Treasurer's down Holborne, the coachman I found to drive easily and easily, at last stood still, and come down hardly able to stand, and told me that he was suddenly struck very sicke, and almost blind, he could not see; so I 'light and went into another coach, with a sad heart for the poor man and troubled for myself, lest

he should have been struck with the plague, being at the end of the towne that I took him up; but God have mercy upon us all!

By the end of June, wagons and people on foot were clogging the roads out of London as people sought safety elsewhere. Pepys finally got his wife Elizabeth away on 5 July, and that night wrote about feeling lonely without her, but added, 'Some trouble there is in having the care of a family at home in this plague time.'

Two weeks later, he noted while on a flying visit to a provincial town that people there shunned refugees from London as having come from the epicentre of the disease: 'Lord! To see, among other things, how all these great people here are afeared of London, being doubtful of anything that comes from thence, or that hath lately been there insomuch that I am troubled at it.' Also in July, the preceding Plague Orders having proven insufficient, Lord Mayor Bloodworth ordered the removal of all dead dogs, cats 'and other vermin' with the destruction of all stray cats and dogs. The official dogcatcher would eventually be praised for killing 4,380 dogs.

A very different style of contemporary diarist was John Evelyn (1620–1706). Born into a wealthy family that had made its money in the manufacture of gunpowder, he travelled on the Continent to avoid taking sides in the civil war between the Parliamentarians and Royalists, which may have been decided outside Oxford by an outbreak of typhus which ravaged both armies, forcing Charles I to abandon his drive on London. Evelyn married Mary, a daughter of the English ambassador in Paris, while on the way home. Together, they had eight children, only one of whom would survive her parents. Evelyn was a founder member of the Royal Society who was driven by insatiable curiosity, and wrote one of the first anti-pollution treatises. Entitled *Fumifugium, or the Inconveniences of the Aer and Smoak of London Dissipated*, it was published in 1661. Three years later, he was appointed one of four Commissioners for Taking Care of Sick and Wounded Seamen and the Care and Treatment of Prisoners of War.

Unlike Pepys, Evelyn did not live in the city of London, but four miles down-river at the separate town of Deptford in a fine property named Sayes Court, adjacent to the navy yard and arsenal. Whereas Pepys crammed into his diary events, thoughts, gossip and scandal,

Evelyn's writing, occasionally using hindsight, was dry and succinct, albeit a trifle pious to modern eyes. On 16 July 1665 he wrote: 'There died of the plague in London this week 1,100 [persons], and in the week following, above 2,000. Two houses were shut up in our parish [of Deptford].'[7]

On 18 July Pepys recorded that 1,089 had died of the plague that week, and deplored burials taking place in plague pits:

> I was much troubled this day to hear at Westminster how the officers do bury the dead in the open Tuttle-fields [he means Tothill Fields in Westminster], pretending want of room elsewhere [when] there [is] still room to be had in at least one of London's cemeteries, and such as are able to pay dear for it, can be buried there.

In late July, Pepys' servant Will suddenly developed a headache. Fearing that his entire house would be shut up if any person came down with the plague, Pepys forced the other servants to throw the man out of the house as quickly as possible. Since Will felt better next day and had no signs of plague, he returned to work, to everyone's great relief.

Although Londoners and people living in the provinces may not have been aware of it, the anti-plague measures taken in Protestant England were determined by justices of the peace for purely rational, if largely unscientific, reasons. On the Catholic continent, however, the situation was clouded by processions bearing holy relics supposedly capable of invoking God's mercy, and by the use of holy water as a supposed disinfectant.

There were however many English pest houses where victims and their families could be confined, to isolate them. After the epidemic of 1603, King James I had ordered pest houses to be established in England; at first only in Oxford, Newcastle and Windsor. In the epidemic of 1625 London had no pest houses as such, just a few hovels in the fields outside the city where sufferers could be locked away. By 1665, however, the city had set aside five pest houses able to accommodate up to 600 victims and all paid for by parish taxes.[8] As already noted, the pest houses were not hospitals, but simply anterooms for death and a way of reducing contact with healthy people. In response to complaints of the treatment of victims' families, in May 1666 Charles II decided to confine in them only the victims and spare their families the humiliation and suffering of being also locked away.[9]

On the Continent, most of the dead were buried by relatives; those from a religious community by fellow monks or nuns. People who died alone often ended up as corpses in the street or in a ditch. What help they may have received toward the end came from monks of mendicant orders like the Capucins. With Henry VIII's abolition of the religious foundations in the late 1530s, in England these functions were taken over by the parishes, who tended to appoint an old woman on a miserly stipend to examine corpses to find the cause of death and notify the appropriate authorities.[10] The system lent itself to abuse; so much so that in 1720 Dr Richard Mead demanded that these 'ignorant old women' should be replaced by 'serious and educated men'.[11]

Pepys assiduously noted that there were no boats on the normally crowded Thames and nobody in the streets, where, following a royal proclamation of 1578, in times of plague fires were kept burning on the pavement or in braziers in the hope of cleansing the air of the miasma or bad air created by rotting organic matter and identifiable by its foul smell, which was thought to be the cause of the plague. There was also an eccentric Quaker named Solomon Eccles or Eagles, said to be a musician, who ran through the streets half-naked with a small brazier of hot coals worn like a hat on his head.[12] In 'The Rules for Preventing the Sickness' published that year in London it was also recommended to cleanse the air in the home with aromatic plants, rose water or vinegar.[13] Used for many purposes, vinegar was also liberally sprayed on the ground above the plague pits; Vinegar Alley in Walthamstow still commemorates the plague pit near St Mary's church.[14]

For its reputed prophylactic powers, Pepys took to chewing tobacco. Others powdered the tobacco and put it into a glass of wine, which they drank and found to be emetic.[15] Similarly, the men paid to cart away the bodies to the plague pits chain-smoked pipes, which left their hands free, trusting in the American weed's reputed powers. Smoking tobacco was made compulsory for all schoolchildren; at Eton, pupils who refused to do so were whipped.[16]

In the diary entry of 26 July one senses Pepys' moment of despair: 'But Lord! To see how the plague spreads.'

On 10 August 1665 he recorded

> an odd story ... of Alderman Bence's stumbling at night
> over a dead corps in the streete, and going home and telling
> his wife, she at the fright, being with child, fell sicke and
> died of the plague.

On 12 August, Pepys wrote:

> My Lord Mayor commands people to be within by 9 at
> night, all (as they say) that the sick may have liberty to go
> abroad for ayre.

On 16 August, he wrote:

> But, Lord! How sad a sight it is to see the streets empty of
> people, and very few upon the 'Change. Jealous [nervous]
> of every door that one sees shut up, lest it should be the
> plague, and about us two shops in three, if not more,
> generally shut up.

On 20 August:

> After to my inn, and eat and drink, and so about seven o'clock
> by water, and got between nine and ten to [Queenhythe],
> very dark. And I could not get my waterman to go [further]
> for fear of the plague.

The watermen, who made a living like modern taxi-drivers by rowing
paying passengers up and down the river, were also vital for anyone
wishing to cross the Thames other than at London bridge, still the only
direct access from the city to the southern suburbs. To an habitual user
of these boats like Pepys, to be deprived of this means of transport was
another inconvenience of the plague. On 22 August he wrote:

> I walked to Greenwich, in my way seeing [an open] coffin
> with a dead body therein, dead of the plague, lying in an
> open close belonging to Coome farme, which was carried

out last night, and the parish have not appointed any body to bury it; but only a watch there day and night, that nobody should go thither or come thence, which is a most cruel thing: this disease making us more cruel to one another than if we are doggs. Saw Bagwell's wife and daughter and went into the daughter's house and *faciebam le cose que ego tenebam in mind con elle.*

The diary entry for 31 August reads:

Thus this month ends, with great sadness upon the publick through the greatness of the plague, everywhere through the Kingdom almost. Every day sadder and sadder news of its encrease. In the City died this week 7,496; and of them 6,102 of the plague. But it is feared that the true number of the dead this week is near 10,000 – partly from the poor that cannot be notice taken of them, and partly from the Quakers and other that will not have any bell ring for them.

In the 2020 outbreak of Covid-19, some people apparently believed that the cause might be 5G connections stimulating the virus. With perhaps greater logic, Pepys changed his mind at least once about buying a new periwig, in case the hair had been taken from a deceased plague victim and might transfer the infection to him.[17] On 3 September 1665, he wrote:

Up, and put on my coloured silk suit very fine, and my new periwigg, bought a good while since, but durst not wear, because the plague was in Westminster when I bought it. It is a wonder what will be the fashion after the plague is done, as to periwiggs, for nobody will dare to buy any haire, for fear of the infection, that it had been cut off of the heads of people dead of the plague.

People were by now terrified of fleas, although Pepys remarked that he did not suffer from them. On one occasion while travelling when he had shared a strange bed with a friend three years before the plague, all the fleas attached themselves to the other man during the night and left

Pepys alone. It is known that fleas dislike certain scents, so a possible reason might be that Pepys used some perfume or cologne which kept them at bay. Most people bitten by a flea never notice the insect discreetly clambering aboard the new host, the species having perfected this crucial manoeuvre over several million years.

Aware of this, agricultural labourers used to tie a string around their trousers below the knee before entering an old barn. Fleas would thus be trapped above the boot and below the string, making them easy to pick off before they had done much biting. Lacking country wisdom, the rest of us only become aware of the arrival of a flea on the following morning, when its bites are showing red and itchy, the sated parasite impossible to punish because it is hiding during daylight between the edge of the fitted carpet of the bedroom and the wall, preparing for the next night's foray and another blood meal. The ability of *pulex irritans* to survive for long periods between feeds was illustrated some years ago when the author visited a house that had not been entered for the better part of a year, and awoke next morning to find the evidence of its presence in a rash of itching red spots.

Among many who had changed sides after the death of Oliver Cromwell was General George Monck (1608–1670), who had been governor of Scotland, but marched his army from there all the way to London, to put an end to the Rump Parliament that governed for a year of confusion. No one had a very high opinion of Monck's intelligence, Edward Hyde, first earl of Clarendon, remarking, 'it is glory enough to his memory that he was instrumental in bringing those things to pass which he had neither the wisdom to foresee, nor courage to attempt, nor understanding to contrive'. For Charles II, however, Monck merited all the honours and senior offices showered upon him, as well as the gift of the territory on the other side of the Atlantic that became North and South Carolina.

What with the war with France and Holland and the plague, England was in a parlous state. On 8 August, Pepys wrote: 'I waited on the Duke of Albemarle [General Monck] He was resolved to stay at the Cockpit, in St James's Park. Died this week in London, 4,000 people.' The duke was one of those who stayed in London, at the King's command. On 15 August, with the plague at its height, Evelyn wrote dryly: 'There perished this week 5,000.' And, on 28 August he added:

The contagion still increasing, and growing now all about us, I sent my wife and whole family (two or three necessary servants excepted) to my brother's at Wotton [a few miles east of Guildford], being resolved to stay at my house myself, and to look after my charge [i.e. carry out the duties of commissioner], trusting in the providence and goodness of God.

Pepys had worked as a clerk in the Exchequer before being persuaded by Lord Sandwich, impressed by this bright young man to whom he was related, mentioning the prospect of bribes if he moved to the Admiralty as its chief secretary charged with victualling the fleet. He lived in a house next to his office in the Admiralty precinct on Seething Lane, west of Tower Hill. Mixing daily with the great and good, including even King Charles II and his brother the Duke of York, also Admiral of the Fleet, he was in a privileged position to hear high-class gossip. By mid-August, he had drawn up his will, writing 'that I shall be in much better state of soul, I hope, if it should please the Lord to call me away this sickly time'.

Later that month, he wrote of deserted streets; the few pedestrians he encountered 'walking like people that had taken leave of the world'.

Chapter 7

The Plague Progresses

London's Company of Parish Clerks was responsible for printing the weekly tallies of burials, known as Bills of Mortality. At the end of August 1665, as the peak of fatalities approached, Pepys noted the latest Bill recording 6,102 victims that week, yet commented that the true number of the week's victims was nearer 10,000, the discrepancy being due to deaths of the urban poor, Catholics and infants not being counted. Adjusting for this omission, historians have estimated the total number of deaths in London as somewhere between 80,000 and 100,000. This, representing a loss of at most 20 per cent of London's population, compares favourably with the 40 to 50 per cent lost in the plague at Barcelona in 1651–53, Naples in 1656 and Genoa in 1657.

A week later, Pepys noted the official number of 6,978 in one week. It was, he wrote, 'a most dreadfull Number'. He was alarmed to note that people attended funerals in spite of official orders to stay at home. Plague victims were supposed to be buried at night, so as not to alarm the general populace, but Pepys complained that burials were taking place in broad daylight, with the tolling of church bells for funerals day and night. Later, no church bells would be rung, but only handbells, as the louder sound worried the sick and those who feared becoming sick. Even then, the iron-shod wheels of the death carts rolling along the cobbled streets, carting off corpses to the mass graves, made the night hideous. The diary noted the deaths of relatives, friends, colleagues, his brewer and baker. The sight of strangers' bodies lying in the street by day was soon so common that he wrote, 'I am almost come to think nothing of it.'

John Evelyn also noted on 7 September 1665:

Came home, there perishing near 10,000 poor creatures weekly; however, I went all along the city and suburbs from Kent Street to St James's, a dismal passage, and dangerous to see so many coffins exposed in the streets, now thin of people; the shops shut up and all in mournful silence, not knowing whose turn might be next. I went to the Duke of Albemarle for a pest-ship, to wait upon our infected men, who were not a few.

On 14 September, Evelyn joined his family in Wotton, but three days later

Receiving a letter from Lord Sandwich of a defeat given to the Dutch, I was forced to travel [home] all Sunday. I was exceedingly perplexed to find that near 3,000 prisoners were sent to me to dispose of, being more than I had places fit to receive and guard.

On 25 September, that prisoner crisis was still unresolved:

My Lord Admiral [the Duke of York] being come from the fleet to Greenwich, I went thence with him to the Cock-pit, to consult with the Duke of Albemarle. I was peremptory that, unless we had £10,000 immediately, the prisoners would starve, and it was proposed that it should be raised out of the [proceeds of the Dutch East India Company] prizes now taken by Lord Sandwich. They being but two of the commission, and so not empowered to determine, sent an express to his Majesty and Council, to know what they should do. In the meantime, I had five vessels, with competent guards, to keep the prisoners in for the present, to be placed as I should think best.

On 28 September, Evelyn went back to Lord Albemarle, to remind him of the deplorable situation, and 'returned with orders'. And so on 29 September:

To Erith, to quicken the sale of the prizes lying there, with order to the commissioner who lay on board till they should be disposed of, £5,000 being proportioned for my quarter. Then I delivered the Dutch Vice-Admiral, who was my prisoner, to Mr Lo[man] of the Marshalsea, he giving me bond in £500 to produce him at my call. I exceedingly pitied this brave unhappy person who had lost with these prizes £40,000 after twenty years' negotiation [i.e. trading] in the East Indies.

There was another reason why Evelyn pitied his Dutch prisoner: the Marshalsea prison in Southwark, south of the Thames, was known for ill-treatment of prisoners and torture, with many dying from their injuries there. On 11 October 1665 Evelyn had to go to London and

> went through the whole city, having occasion to alight out of the coach in several places about business of money, when I was environed with multitudes of poor, pestiferous creatures begging alms; the shops universally shut up, a dreadful prospect! I dined with my Lord General [Monck], was to receive £10,000, and had guards to convey both myself and it, and so returned home through God's infinite mercy.

Evelyn was 45 years old on 31 October, for which he also thanked God's infinite mercy. At the end of November, he noted that the contagion had decreased considerably, but on New Year's Eve he wrote:

> Now blessed be God, for his extraordinary mercies and preservation of me this year, when thousands, and ten thousands, perished and were swept away on each side of me, there dying in our parish [of Deptford] 406 of the pestilence!

Daniel Defoe – born Daniel Foe, adding the aristocratic French prefix De when adult – had a varied career, being at various times a hosier, wine merchant, spy, poet, traveller, economist and novelist. Coming from a family of Dissenters, he was denied entrance to schools and universities, thereby lacking the Classics and being tutored in such new subjects as astronomy and geography. While in jail for debt, he wrote *An Essay upon Projects*, proposing a central bank, income tax and a commission to check evasion, plus life and health insurance for sailors and soldiers, toll roads, the direction of labour, the building of a national road network, a military academy and women's rights.[1] This was all revolutionary stuff. In 1703 Defoe was placed in stocks as a public punishment and satirised the event with *A Hymn to the Pillory*. It was his satire on Anglican discrimination against Dissenters that saw him jailed in Newgate prison 'during Her Majesty's pleasure' for seditious libel. With his wife and seven children near starvation, Defoe humbled himself and, with the help of a Tory politician and the lord treasurer, secured his release.[2] He also did his homework for his book *A Journal of the Plague Year*, published in 1722, and listed the Orders Conceived and Published by the Lord Mayor and Aldermen of the City of London concerning the Infection of the Plague in August 1665. These included:

Examiners to be appointed in every Parish
In every Parish, there be one, two, or more Persons of good Sort and Credit, chosen and appointed by the Alderman, his Deputy, and common-Council of every Ward, by the Name of Examiners, to continue in that Office the Space of two Months at least: And if any fit Person so appointed, shall refuse to undertake the same ... [they shall be] committed to Prison until they shall conform themselves accordingly.

The Examiners Office
And if they find any Person sick of the Infection, to give order to the Constable that the House be shut up; and if the Constable shall be found Remiss or Negligent, to give present Notice thereof to the Alderman of the Ward.

Watchmen
THAT to every infected House there be appointed two Watchmen, one for every day, and the other for the Night. And that these Watchmen have a special care that no Person go in or out of such infected Houses, whereof they have the Charge, upon pain of severe Punishment.

Searchers
THAT there be a special care to appoint Women-Searchers in every Parish, such as are of honest Reputation, and of the best Sort as can be got in this kind: And these to be

sworn to make due Search, and true Report to the utmost of their Knowledge, whether the Persons whose bodies they are appointed to Search, do die of the Infection, or what other Disease as near as they can. And that the Physicians who shall be appointed ... do call before them the said Searchers ... that they may consider, whether they are fitly qualified for that Employment, and charge them if they shall see Cause, if they appear defective in their Duties.

Chirurgeons

FOR better assistance of the Searchers ... that there be chosen and appointed able and discreet Chirurgeons ... and the said Chirurgeons ... to join with the Searchers for the View of the Body, to the end that there may be a true Report made of the Disease.

It is ordered that every one of the said Chirurgeons shall have Twelvepence a Body searched by them, to be paid out of the Goods of the Party searched, if he be able, or otherwise by the Parish.

The *Orders Concerning Infected Houses, and Persons Sick of the Plague,* published at the same time, also covered how notice was to be given of the sickness by 'the Master of the House' and the sequestration of the sick person or persons. The section entitled *Airing the Stuff* specified how the bed linen, curtains and clothes of the deceased person must be well aired 'with Fire' and that no items were to be carried out of the infected house or sold off for twenty days after the death of the former owner. The section headed *Shutting up of the House* gave the examiner the power of deciding for how long an infected house must remain closed and unused. *Burial of the Dead* specified at what time a burial could be made and how many adults could be present, children being excluded. *Every Visited House to be Marked* listed the markings on the door of a house visited by the plague, to warn people off. *Every Visited House to be Watched* listed in detail how an infected house should be closely watched and by whom. There was even one section entitled *Hackney-Coaches* which punished each driver who had carried a sufferer to the pest-house by losing the use of his coach for five or six days afterward, when it had been thoroughly aired.

The *Orders for Cleansing and Keeping of the Streets Sweet* made it the responsibility of each householder to sweep and keep clean the street in front of his house, the sweepings to be carried away daily by the rakers who, in normal times, had the unpleasant duty of removing excrement from the street. No laystalls or deposits of dung were to be allowed in the City, and no stinking 'Fish or unwholesome Flesh or musty Corn, or other corrupt Fruits' be sold there. Separately, it was ordained 'That no Hogs, Dogs or Cats or tame Pigeons or Conies [rabbits]' be kept within any part of the City. Dogs were to be killed by the dog-killers and any stray swine to be impounded by the Beadle and the owner punished according to the Act of Common-Council.

> The last ordinance proclaimed that the City had no wandring Beggers ... being a great cause of the spreading of the Infection ... be suffered in the Streets of this City under threat of dire penalty. All Plays, Bear-Baitings, singing of Ballads, Buckler-play or such like Causes of Assemblies of People [were] utterly prohibited as [were] all publick Feasting ... and dinners at Taverns, Alehouses and other Places of common Entertainment.

The idea was that the money thus saved could be preserved and employed for the relief of the poor. Finally, 'disorderly Tipling in Taverns, Ale-houses, Coffe-Houses and cellars [was to] be severely looked into [and the said establishments to close at 9 p.m.]'.[3]

Also in August, Defoe was cautioned by his friend Dr Heath against going outside the house, but to lock himself and his family up and keep the windows and shutters closed and curtains drawn, only opening them after making 'a very strong Smoke with Rozen and Pitch, Brimstone or Gunpowder in the Room where the Window or Door was to be opened.' This was intended to counter the plague-bearing miasma.[4]

It was all very well for the good doctor to advise but, with no store of food in the house, it was necessary for Defoe to go out shopping. Although he commented on the Assize of Bread keeping the price of bread pretty stable despite panic buying, and with many bakers still working normally, Defoe avoided bakeries, fearing that they were plague foci with all the servants standing around waiting for their masters' dough to be baked.[5] He preferred to buy flour, with which to bake bread for the family, as well as salted butter, cheese, and malt, to brew beer. Meat, however, was not safely to be found, too many butchers being infected. Venturing into any market was risky, as Defoe observed:

> Sometimes a Man or Woman dropt down Dead in the very Markets; for many People that had the Plague upon them, knew nothing of it; till the inward Gangreen had affected their Vitals and they dy'd in a few Moments; this caused that many died frequently in that Manner in the Streets suddainly, without any warning: Others perhaps had Time to go to the next Bulk or Stall [in front of a shop]; or to any Door, Porch, and just sit down and die.[6]

By mid-September of 1665 people paid less attention to the quarantine rules requiring social distancing. Shades of Britain in 2020! Gentlemen recommenced gathering in places like the Royal Exchange, where they were wont to make deals and catch up on the gossip in an adjacent coffee-shop. Pepys was one of them. As the plague peaked with 8,000 deaths in London during one week, he wrote of enjoying a good drink with his friend Captain Cocke. Alcohol, then as now, met the needs of the moment. As Pepys put it, 'I am fain to allow [it to] myself during this plague time, my physician being dead.'

On 24 September, he wrote:

> In this sad time of the plague every thing else has conspired to my happiness and pleasure more for these last three months than in all my life ... May God preserve it and make me thankful for it.

The note of 7 October included how he had 'come close by the bearers with a dead corpse of the plague, but Lord, to see what custom is, that I am come almost to think nothing of it.' That month, lust got the better of prudence. He visited a lady friend, although 'round about and next door on every side is the plague, but I did not value it but there did what I could *con ella*'.

On 16 October, he laments:

> I walked to the Tower. But Lord! How empty the streets are
> and melancholy, so many poor sick people in the streets
> full of sores; and so many sad stories overheard as I walk,
> everybody talking of this dead, and that man sick. They tell
> me that in Westminster there is never a physician and but
> one apothecary left, all being dead, but that there are great
> hopes of a great decrease [in cases] this week: God send it!

Most people in need of treatment went to a barber-surgeon, apothecary
or healer, more accessible and cheaper than doctors, or simply self-
medicated using traditional, mainly herbal, medicine.[7] Three of the
king's physicians remained in London throughout the plague by royal
command, in theory to care for the poor, who could not afford to pay a
doctor's fee. All three, it seems, survived.[8] One doctor worthy of note
in the London College of Physicians was Nathaniel Hodges (1629–
1688). In 1665 he was co-opted onto an emergency committee: himself
and one other doctor, plus two municipal councillors and two sheriffs.
He accepted that the available medical knowledge could do nothing to
halt the epidemic, instead recommending quarantine measures with
severe penalties for infringement and forbidding dangerous or deadly
quack drugs taken as reputed cures.

In 1672 he published his observations, firstly in Latin, which every
other doctor could read without the common people understanding it,
and then in English with the magnificent title *Loimologia, or a Historical
Account of the Plague in London; with Precautionary Direction against
the like Contagion*. In it, Hodges did his best to unite the Galenian theory
of humours, the theory that miasmas produced plague and the work of
Athanasius Kircher, who said he had seen minute forms of life in blood
samples from plague victims. In ignoring astrology, folk myths and
superstitions inculcated by panic, his book was a considerable advance
on previous writings.[9] In 1720 it was re-published in French during the
plague of Marseilles, and was freely used by Daniel Defoe when he
came to write *A Journal of the Plague Year* in 1722.[10]

Another attempt to remove medical practice from the realms of
hearsay and superstition was made by Robert Boyle (1627–1691),
an Anglo-Irish Old Etonian, son of the immensely rich earl of Cork.

Boyle was both a chemist and an experimental physicist. Elected a member of the newly founded Royal Society for the Improvement of Natural Knowledge, he is today best known for originating Boyle's Law of gases.[11] His impoverished assistant Robert Hooke FRS (1635–1703), who made most of Boyle's experimental apparatus, invented a microscope through which he could clearly see microorganisms living in blood samples. In turn, this enabled Boyle to formulate the hypothesis that microscopically small corpuscles exuded from plague victims could penetrate the skin of healthy people and infect them – a process that could be blocked by treating their skin. Hooke drew accurate and exquisitely detailed enlarged representations of a flea and a louse. His microscopic examination of fossils and logical deductions of their age, made him a precursor of Darwin. A genuine polymath, later deservedly enriched by his own genius, Hooke also invented a telescope enabling him to observe Mars and Jupiter, and to map craters on the moon.

Dr Thomas Sydenham (1624–1689) was the most celebrated medical man in England at the time of the great plague. Licensed to practise medicine in and around Westminster, he stayed for a while to treat victims, but then fled to the country with his family, later being among the earliest returnees. His experience-based account *metodus curandi febres* or *The Method of Curing Fevers Based on His Own Observations* was published in 1666. He too rejected any astrological causes of the plague, but blamed miasmas for changing the quality of the air. This could be combated, he believed, by purging, sweating and bleeding, all of which processes he claimed to have successfully tried himself. Although correctly distinguishing several types of fever he had observed, he wrongly concluded that in an epidemic they all merged into the dominant malady.[12] Due to his high standing and original thinking, this belief persisted in England until the end of the nineteenth century.

Founded in 1518, the London College of Physicians had fifty licensed doctors at the time of the plague. In addition, the barber-surgeons, who monopolised cutting because they possessed sharp blades and bled the sick, numbered as many as 100, and there were 100 apothecaries and some 250 nurses and midwives of varying capabilities.[13] Although female doctors practised in southern France and in enlightened Italian cities, including Naples and Venice, they were not normally allowed to practise in England, but only during emergencies like the plague. Afterwards, they were forbidden to concern themselves with anything outside midwifery and children's illnesses, in case they were witches intent on casting spells on their patients.[14]

Influenced by the Hippocratic theory of the four humours, doctors in England prescribed 'hot' substances like garlic and ginger, 'cold' substances like vinegar and cucumber and both humidifying and drying treatments in closely guarded recipes.[15] There was also the all-purpose *theriac*, invented by Galen fourteen centuries earlier, being a compound of seventy-four ingredients including snake venom, which was reputed to cure a viper's bite and that of a rabid dog. Prescribed for Roman emperors with unknown results, it came to fame during the plague, with *theriac* made in Venice and Montpellier reputedly the most efficacious. In 1626 the London College of Physicians did away with snake venom in its recipe and upped the dose of opium.[16]

However, if purging, bleeding and cauterisation did not drive the plague out of a sufferer, the College recommended plucking the neck of a living chicken or pigeon and placing the bird's anus on a bubo, to suck up the poison. Ointments made from ingredients as curious as toad's excrement and the poisons arsenic and antimony were also rubbed on the patient's skin or, in dried form, suspended in a small sachet on a cord around the neck.[17] Many useless quack remedies were protected by the 1624 Statute of Monopolies, which prohibited publication of their ingredients. These included Anderson's Scots Pills and the charmingly named Duchess of Kent's Powder, which was equally a waste of money. But some people will try anything in an emergency: during the plague at Marseille in 1720 the French regent Philippe d'Orléans used his own money to manufacture one of these reputed treatments and distribute the pills, which had no effect.

On 15 November 1665, the London Bill of Mortality reported that only 1,300 people had died of the plague that week. This was less than a quarter of the weekly figure a few weeks earlier. The next Bill halved that figure for the following week, reporting only 600 people dead. People attributed this to the winter's first real frost.

On 24 November Pepys found the Royal Exchange crowded with men he knew making deals, quite like old times. So much so that he and Elizabeth started discussing their move back to the house in London. During the outbreak, Pepys had been very concerned with his frame of mind; he frequently mentioned trying to be in good spirits. The Hippocratic theory of four humours – blood, phlegm, yellow bile and black bile – having to be in balance for one's health still held sway. If a patient had fever, the doctor prescribed bleeding to reduce the temperature. The same theory blamed depression on an excess of black bile. So, when hearing of friends and acquaintances who had died, Pepys endeavoured to block his natural sadness and look on the bright side. But, on 13 December 1665, the reality was:

> The plague is encreased again this week, notwithstanding there hath been a day or two great frosts, but we hope it is only the effects of the late close, warm weather and, if the frosts continue the next week, may fall again

One can forgive seventeenth-century people having their superstitions in the absence of scientific education. As autumn became winter, they told themselves that the colder weather would see the epidemic taper off and die out. Yet in the Covid-19 pandemic there were similar fake epidemiologists, like US President Trump, who announced early in 2020 that the virus would disappear when temperatures rose with the advent of summer weather, and suggested swallowing domestic cleaning products to kill the coronavirus. Pepys was less gullible: when a noble patroness gave him a bottle of plague water – a concoction of several herbs reputed to be a certain cure – he was rightly sceptical. Having participated in a coffee-house discussion about the plague increasing in London and possible remedies against it, he commented that all was just opinion and equally unfounded.

With a third of London's population, estimated at 420,000 before the plague, having died, on 31 December 1665 Pepys recorded:

> The plague is abated almost to nothing. But many of such as I know very well, dead. Yet, to our great joy, the town fills apace and shops begin to be open again. Pray God continue the plague's decrease! for that keeps the Court away from the place of business, and so all goes to rack as to publick matters, they at this distance not thinking of it.

Two months later, it was considered safe for King Charles II and the court to return to the capital, although cases of plague continued to be noted in towns as far apart as Nottingham and Winchester in 1667 and 1668.

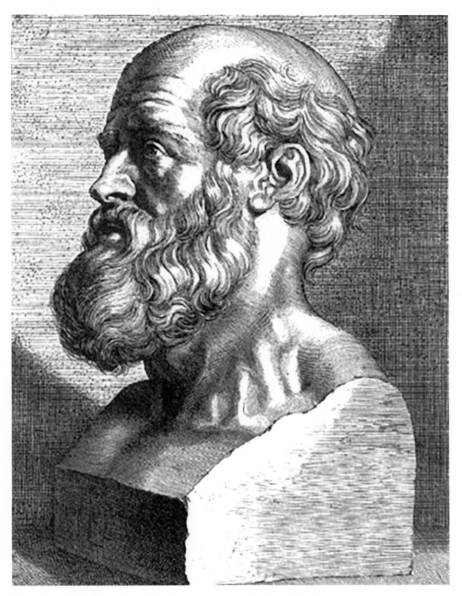

The Greek philosopher Hippocrates recognised epidemics and pandemics more than 2,000 years ago. He had only his own intelligence to work with. Today, science has made tools to travel into space and visit other planets, yet a pandemic can appear out of nowhere and take the whole human race by surprise. Makes you think, doesn't it?

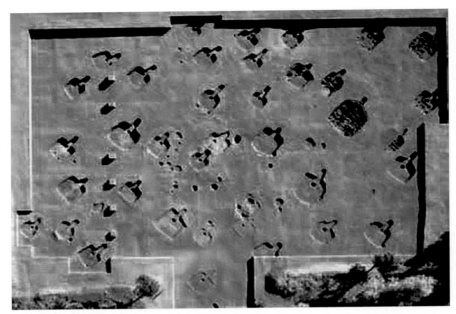

Many prehistoric cities were mysteriously abandoned undamaged. So was the Neolithic settlement of Hamin Manga in Mongolia 5,000 years ago (aerial view of excavations above). Only a plague outbreak can explain the inhabitants' sudden flight. In the Toggenburg Bible of 1411, the Egyptian plague of boils is depicted (below). Was this bubonic plague, or smallpox?

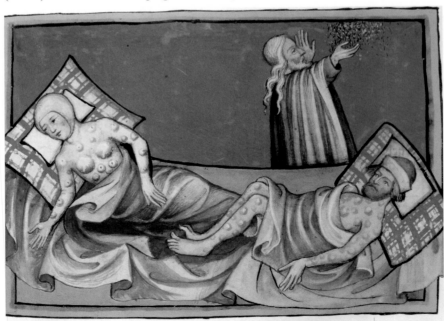

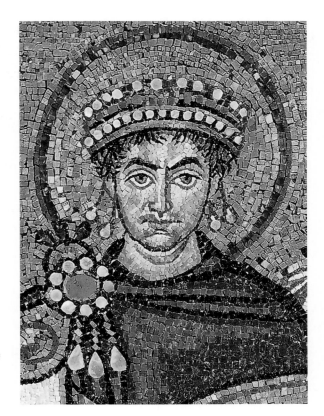

A bubonic plague swept the eastern Roman Empire of Justinian I (portrait in mosaic right), claiming several thousand lives *each day* inside the walls of Constantinople. And plague is still with us (see WHO map below)

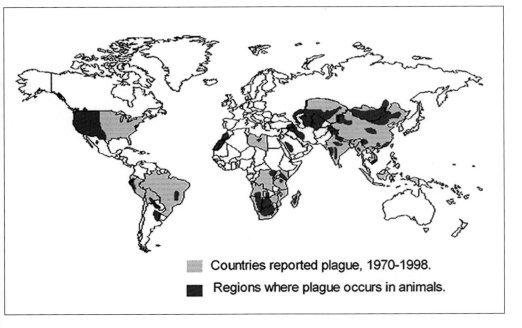

Countries reported plague, 1970-1998.

Regions where plague occurs in animals.

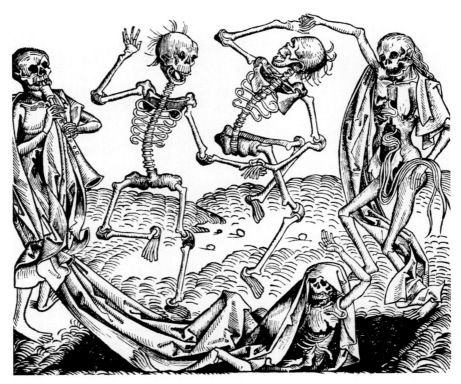

In the Nuremburg Chronicle c. 1493 artist Michael Wolgemut memorialised plague victims in his Dance of the Skeletons (above). He also depicted the burning alive of Jews, blamed for the plague by Christians (below).

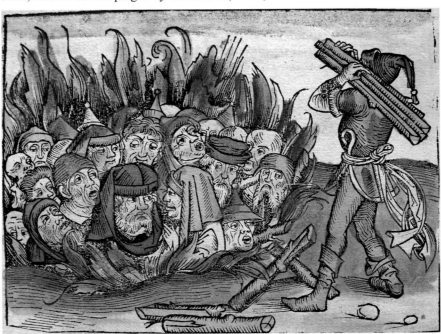

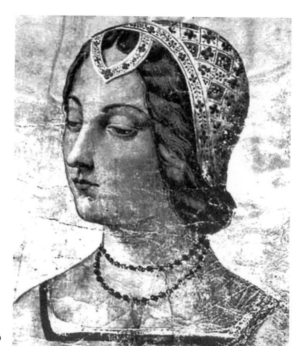

When his beloved Laura
(above) died in 1348, the
poet of the plague Francisco
Petrarca (below) wrote
'death looked lovely in her
face'. This proved he never
saw her dead, for plague
victims did *not* look lovely.

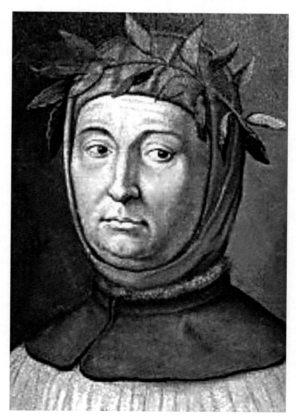

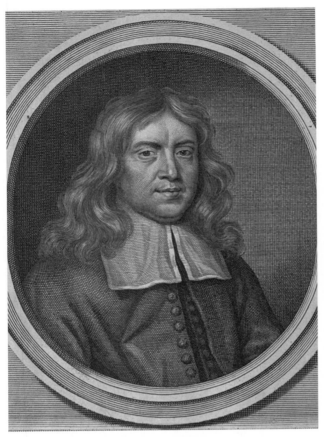

Most of what we know of London's Black Death comes from these four men. Thomas Sydenham (left) wrote *Observationes medicae,* used as a textbook for more than a century afterwards.

Prolific diarist Samuel Pepys (below, right) had to keep working in London throughout the plague. His contemporary John Evelyn (below, left), lived less dangerously down-river at Deptford.

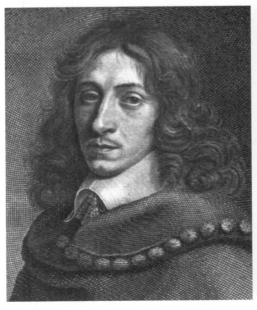

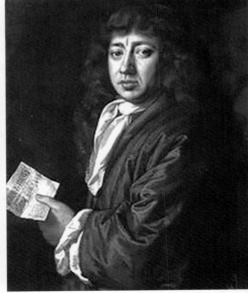

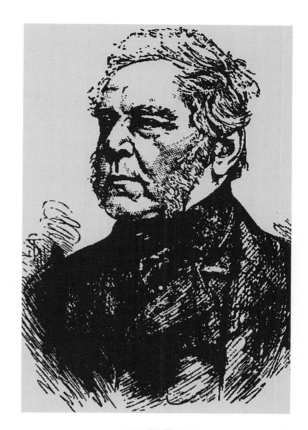

Every week the parish clerks drew up Bills of Mortality (below) but haberdasher John Graunt (above) was also a pioneer demographer and epidemiologist. He thought they under-estimated.

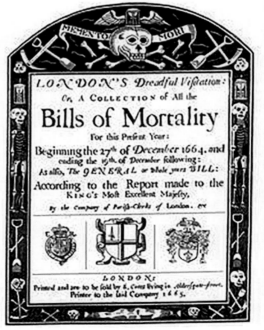

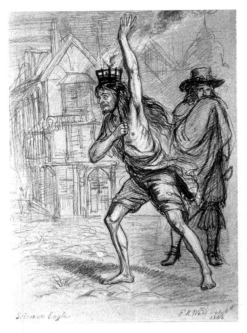

Solomon Eagle   E.M.Ward Sculpsit 1864

During the Great Plague of 1665–6, fires were lit in London streets to drive away the 'bad air' thought to cause the sickness and a Quaker named Solomon Eagles ran everywhere with a brazier of burning coals on his head (left). A few brave physicians dissected plague corpses (below), but they could not see the cause.

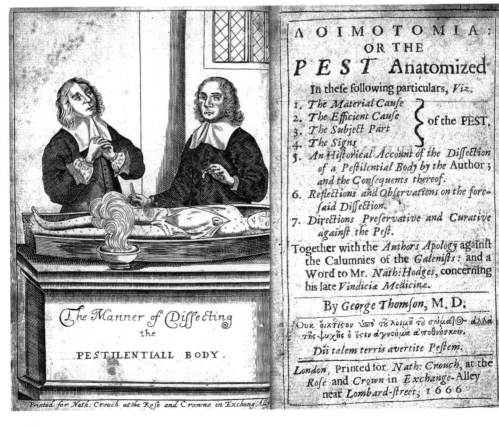

The Manner of Dissecting the PESTILENTIALL BODY.

Printed for Nath: Crouch at the Rose and Crowne in Exchang Ally

ΛΟΙΜΟΤΟΜΙΑ:
OR THE
PEST Anatomized

In these following particulars, Viz.

1. The Material Cause
2. The Efficient Cause   } of the PEST.
3. The Subject Part
4. The Signs
5. An Historical Account of the Dissection of a Pestilential Body by the Author; and the Consequents thereof.
6. Reflections and Observations on the foresaid Dissection.
7. Directions Preservative and Curative against the Pest.

Together with the Authors Apology against the Calumnies of the Galenists: and a Word to Mr. Nath: Hodges, concerning his late Vindiciæ Medicinæ.

By George Thomson, M.D.

Οὐκ οἰκτιστὸν ὑπὸ τῶ λοιμῶ τὸ σῶμα]Θ- ἀλλὰ τῆς ψυχῆς ὅ ἐστιν ἀγνοήμα ἀποθνήσκειν.

Dii talem terris avertite Pestem.

London, Printed for Nath: Crouch, at the Rose and Crown in Exchange-Alley near Lombard-street, 1666

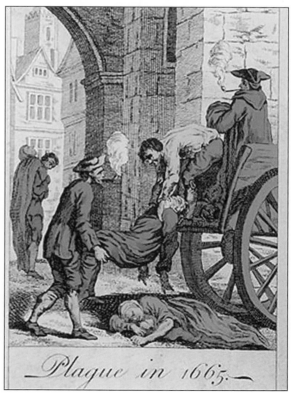

Plague doctors protected themselves as best they could (above). The beak of the face mask was filled with scented herbs to block the odour of death and putrefaction

'Bring out your dead,' they cried and loaded the corpses onto the death carts, (below) tipping their loads into mass graves. Thinking tobacco was a disinfectant, the death cart men smoked all day long.

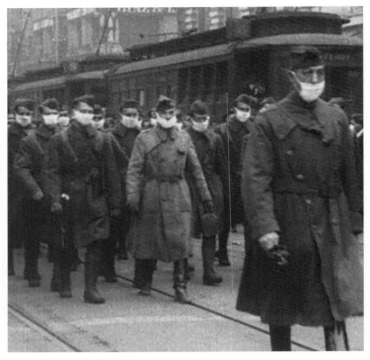

As World War I drew to a close in 1918 an even worse killer surfaced. The 'Spanish flu' did not begin in Spain, but probably in Kansas at Camp Funston, where hundreds of men fell sick (below). Marched to board troopships heading for the trenches in France (above), the survivors brought the virus with them, so that it spread throughout the world.

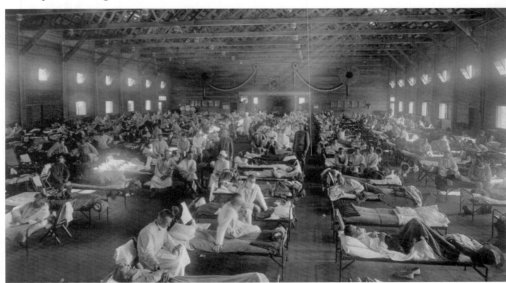

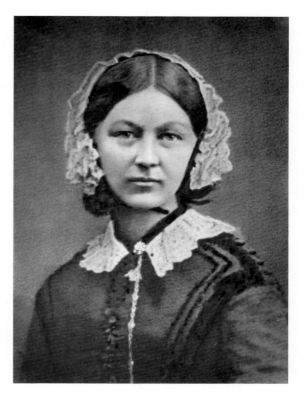

In the Crimean war Florence Nightingale (right) nursed wounded soldiers with dysentery and cholera, bringing the fatalities down from 44 per cent to 2.2 per cent by elementary hygiene. Women also nursed the wounded during World War I and the Spanish flu (below). Many of them died in this pandemic that killed an estimated 100 million people worldwide.

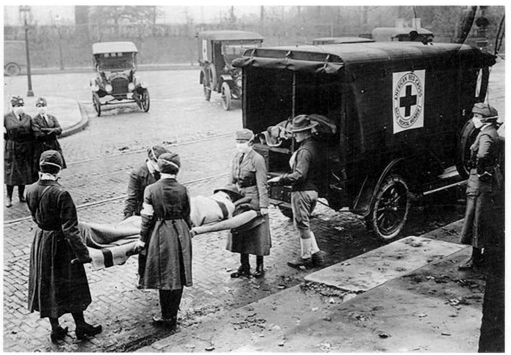

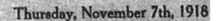

CORPORATION OF THE CITY OF KELOWNA

PUBLIC NOTICE

Notice is hereby given that, in order to prevent the spread of Spanish Influenza, all Schools, public and private, Churches, Theatres, Moving Picture Halls, Pool Rooms and other places of amusement, and Lodge meetings, are to be closed until further notice.

All public gatherings consisting of ten or more are prohibited.

D. W. SUTHERLAND,
Mayor.

Kelowna, B.C.,
19th October, 1918.

In the Covid-19 pandemic, the authorities could not improve on the measures announced by this British Columbian mayor a century earlier (above). Who was then in the audience when these four grotesquely masked and helmeted girls were dancing (below)?

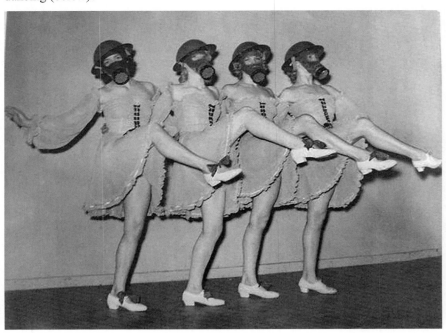

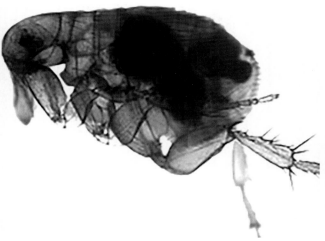

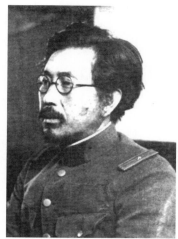

Biological warfare is not new but Surgeon-General Shiro Ishii (above right) took it to new depths in Manchuria after the Japanese invasion of 1931. In his secret death factory at Harbin (below), his men killed 10,000 prisoners in experiments and about a half-million Chinese civilians by air-dropping fleas infected with plague (above left) on their towns.

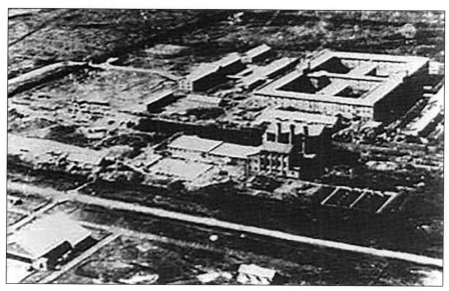

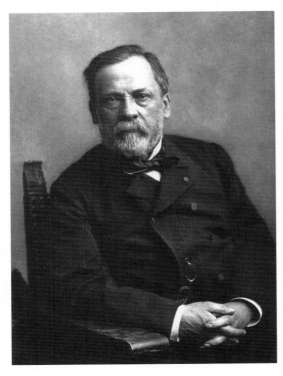

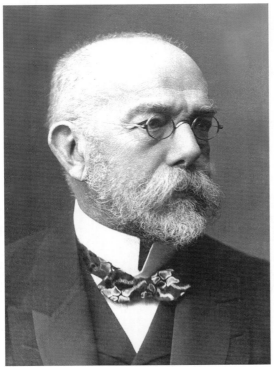

The nineteenth century saw great strides made in the fight against disease and infection. Two of the most famous names in the field are Frenchman Louis Pasteur (above) and German Robert Koch (below).

Each of these three men also saved *millions* of lives. Waldemar Haffkine (right) was a Russian-born zoologist who defied the British government of India and produced successful vaccines for cholera and plague. Also in India, a British army medical officer with a mind of his own was Dr Ronald Ross (below left), who discovered that female anopheles mosquitoes transmitted malaria to humans.

Equally obstinate, Swiss researcher Alexandre Yersin (below right) defied authority in both Hong Kong and London, correctly identifying the bacterium that causes bubonic plague.

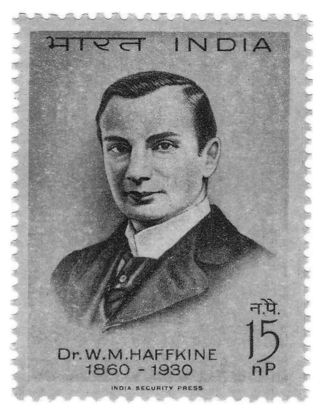

भारत INDIA

Dr. W. M. HAFFKINE
1860 - 1930

INDIA SECURITY PRESS

न.पै.
15
nP

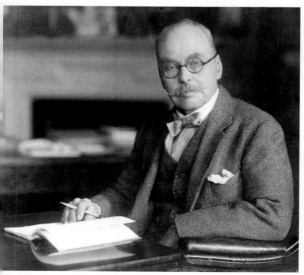

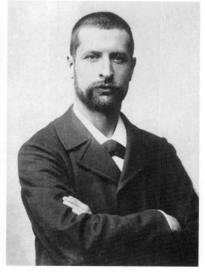

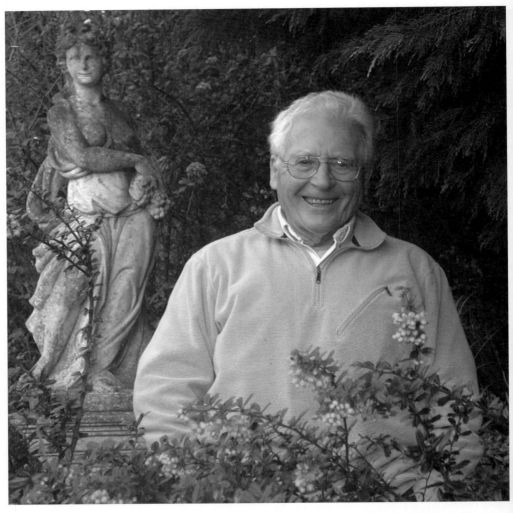

Seen here in his garden is the highly respected scientist, inventor and philosopher James Lovelock CH, FRS, and with a string of other honours and qualifications to his name. Way back in the 1960s, he propounded a hypothesis that our world was a living entity, which he named Gaia after the Greek earth goddess. Epidemics and pandemics can be seen as Gaia's weapons to protect itself against the human species which is destroying the planet. Not everyone agrees with Lovelock, but many influential scientists do.

Chapter 8

Death Goes on Regardless

On 9 January 1666 Pepys noted:

> Up, and then to the office, where we met first since the
> plague, which God preserve us in!

Yet, on the following day, his mood changed:

> To the 'Change, and there hear to our grief how the plague
> is encreased this week from seventy to eighty-nine.

On 12 January 1666 John Evelyn noted:

> After much, and indeed extraordinary mirth and cheer,
> all my brothers, our wives, and children, being together,
> and after much sorrow and trouble during this contagion,
> which separated our families as well as others, I returned
> to my house [in Deptford], but my wife went back
> to Wotton. I, not as yet willing to adventure her, the
> contagion, though exceedingly abated, not as yet wholly
> extinguished among us.

On 13 January Pepys wrote:

> Home with his Lordship to Mrs Williams's, in Covent
> Garden, to dinner (the first time I ever was there) and there
> met Captain Cocke; and pretty merry, though not perfectly
> so, because of the fear that there is of a great encrease again
> of the plague this week. Besides, if the plague continues
> among us another yeare, the Lord knows what will become
> of us.

On 29 January 1666 John Evelyn went to wait on the king, the court being lately returned from Oxford to Hampton Court

> where the Duke of Albemarle presented me to him; he ran toward me, and in a most gracious manner gave me his hand to kiss, with many thanks for my care and faithfulness in his service in a time of such great danger, when everybody fled their appointments; he told me he was very much obliged to me and said he was several times concerned for me, and the peril I underwent and did receive my service most acceptably (though in truth I did but do my duty and O that I had performed it as I ought!). Then the Duke came toward me, and embraced me with much kindness, telling me if he had thought my danger would have been so great, he would not have suffered his Majesty to apply me in that station.

On 13 February Pepys recorded,

> Ill newes this night that the plague is encreased this week and in many places else about the town and at Chatham and elsewhere.

Neverthleess, the Royal Society of learned men reassembled on 22 March 1666, judging it safe to return to London. Down-river at Deptford, John Evelyn recorded a week earlier:

> Our parish was now more infected with the plague than ever, and so was all the country about, though almost quite ceased at London.

On 25 April, Pepys noted that the plague mortality was reduced in London to sixteen that week. By early June, his mood had changed, and on 10 June he showed more interest in high society tittle-tattle than the plague:

> The Duke of York is wholly given up to his new mistress, my Lady Denham, going at noon today with all his gentlemen to visit her in Scotland Yard; she declaring she will not be his

mistress, as Mrs Price, to go up and down the Privy stairs, but will be owned publicly; and so she is. Mr Bruncker, it seems, was the pimp to bring it about, and my Lady Castlemaine, who designed thereby to fortify herself with the Duke; there being a falling-out the other day between the King and her: on this occasion the Queene in ordinary talke between the ladies in her drawing- room, did say to my Lady Castlemaine that she feared the King did take cold, by staying so late abroad at her house. She answered before them all, that he did not stay so late abroad with her, for he went betimes thence (though he do not before one, two or three in the morning) but must stay somewhere else. The King then coming in and overhearing, did whisper in the eare aside, and told her she was a bold impertinent woman, and bid her be gone out of the Court, and not come again till he sent for her, which she did presently, and went to a lodging in the Pell Mell, and kept there two or three days, and then sent to the King to know whether she might send for her things away out of her house. The King sent to her, she must first come and view them, and so she come, and the King went to her, and all friends again. She did, in her anger, say she would be even with the King, and [publish] his letters to her.

In May 1666 the population of Eyam in Derbyshire self-isolated heroically. The story went that, after a parcel of cloth from London was delivered to the two-story cottage of local tailor Alexander Hadfield, his assistant George Viccars noticed that it was damp and unwrapped it. Viccars was not a native of Eyam, but had come there to make clothes for the Wakes Week of 1665 – and was never to leave. He hung the cloth up near a fire, to dry it, and seemingly revived some infected fleas in the parcel. He was among the first victims; between September and December 1665 forty-two other people died in Eyam, leaving the survivors nervously planning their escape to other parts.

Fleas in bundles of cloth have also been suggested as the route by which infected fleas reached east Africa from Gujarat in the early to mid-nineteenth century. Indian merchants shipped the bundles to Zanzibar and sold them to Arab merchants, who had the carried by porters far into the interior.[1]

In Eyam, the new and unpopular rector William Mompesson decided that the village must isolate itself, to prevent the plague being carried to neighbouring villages. He had been appointed to replace the previous incumbent Thomas Stanley, dismissed because he refused to acknowledge the Act of Conformity and use Charles II's *Book of Common Prayer.* Whatever their feelings about each other, Mompesson and Stanley agreed that it was their Christian duty to halt the spread of the plague by persuading the villagers to stay in Eyam, come what may.

A cordon was drawn around the village. The church was closed, Mompesson preaching on a limestone outcrop nearby known as Cucklett Delf with his listeners standing well separated on the opposing hillside across a small stream. The Duke of Devonshire, living nearby at Chatsworth House, arranged for provisions and food to be supplied, for which the villagers paid by placing money, 'sterilised' by immersion in vinegar, on a boundary stone where the supplies were left. This was common practise all over England, the stones with a hollow on the top where payment could be left in a pool of vinegar being referred to as 'plague stones'. An alternative was to leave coins in the running water of a stream, on the bank of which goods could be left.

One example of the suffering that the villagers of Eyam underwent for their faith was that of Elizabeth Hancock, who watched her husband and six children die of the plague in one week and had to drag the bodies into a field, where the village gravedigger Marshall Howe had dug graves, and there bury them herself. Despite handling many of the plague dead, Howe survived, as did Elizabeth Hancock. Possibly, their blood groups were more resistant than those of the dead. Some modern researchers believe that the percentage of Europeans with blood group O is lower than on other continents, and tentatively conclude that this may be because people of the O group were more vulnerable to the plague, so that this blood group was nearly extinguished in the seventeenth century. The self-sacrifice of the 350 inhabitants of Eyam was heroic, costing the lives of 273 villagers,[2] possibly because transmission changed from rats-fleas-humans to pneumonic plague with direct person-to-person contagion. It had in any case no effect on the spread of the disease elsewhere.[3] Villages all over England lost between 40 and 75 per cent of their inhabitants.

Well, that is a marvellous story of Christian self-abnegation, but there are other versions of what happened in Eyam, one of which may be true. On 13 June 1666, Pepys wrote he

> walked to Mrs Bagwell's house, and there (it being by this time pretty dark and past ten o'clock) went into her house and did what I would. But I was not a little fearfull of what she told me, which is, that her servant was dead of the plague, that her coming to me yesterday was the first day of her coming forth [after the forty days of isolation] and that she had new whitened the house all below stairs [with lime-wash as a disinfectant], but that above stairs they are not fit [safe] for me to go up.

On 19 June, Pepys' dalliances blot out both the plague and the recent defeat of the fleet by the Dutch:

> Thence home, and at my business till late at night, then with my wife into the garden and there sang with [the maid] Mercer, whom I feel myself begin to love too much by handling of her breasts of a morning when she dresses me, they being the finest that I ever saw in my life, that is the truth of it. To supper with beans and bacon and to bed.

On 22 June:

> At noon to the 'Change and Coffee-house, where great talke of the Dutch preparing of sixty sayle of ships. The plague grows mightily among them, both at sea and land.

On 4 July he was thanking God that there were only two fatalities in London that week, yet plague was still in Colchester 'where it has long been, and is believed will quite depopulate the place'.

The war with the Dutch was also having an effect on the London streets. On 6 July Pepys commented:

> But it is a pretty thing to observe that a man shall see many women now-a-days of mean sort in the streets, but no men; men being still so afeared of the press [gangs].

On 22 July, John Evelyn recorded that Deptford was still infected with the contagion. And, on 6 August Pepys was worried again:

> In Fenchurche-streete met with Mr Battersby; says he, 'Do you see Dan Rawlinson's door shut up?' (which I did, and wondered) 'Why,' says he, 'After all the sickness, and himself spending all the last year in the country, one of his men is now dead of the plague, and his wife and one of his mayds sicke, and himself shut up,' which troubles me mightily. So home and there do hear also from Mrs Sarah Daniel, that Greenwich is at this time much worse than it ever was, and Deptford too, and she told us that [many people] would come to London; which is now the receptacle of all the people from all infected places. God preserve us.

Three days later:

> In my [way] I inquired, and find Mrs Rawlinson is dead of the sickness, and her mayde continues mighty ill. [Mr Rawlinson] is got out of the house. I met also with Mr Evelyn in the streete, who tells me of the sad condition at this very day at Deptford for the plague, and more at Deale (within his precinct as one of the Commissioners for sick and wounded seamen), that the town is almost quite depopulated. And hear in Fanchurch-Streete that the mayde is also dead at Mr Rawlinson's; so that there are three dead in all, the wife, a man-servant and mayde-servant.

The plague at Deptford continued to the end of August, as we know from John Evelyn's diary. Ironically, given the disaster that was soon to befall London, on 27 August Evelyn was at St Paul's discussing with Christopher Wren and others 'the decay of that ancient and venerable church, and to set down in writing the particulars of what was fit to be done'. The day was wasted because, six days later at about 10 p.m. began the Great Fire.

It is estimated that the population of England was about 5.25 million in 1650; by 1680 it had fallen to 4.9 million. Counting up the Bills of Mortality gives a figure of 68,956 deaths in London but, as with the early figures for Covid-19 in 2020, this is thought to be an under-estimate, excluding non-Protestants and infants, with the true figure nearer to 80,000 or even 100,000.[4] London soon made up for the plague deaths by immigration of the rural poor, so that the population reached 490,000 by 1700. Similarly, Barcelona, badly affected by its plague in 1651–53, Marseilles in 1720, Ukraine in 1737, Messina in 1743 and even Moscow in 1770–71 all swiftly replaced their dead inhabitants.[5] The movement from country to large towns, however, caused the decline and disappearance of many villages and small towns.[6]

Keeping the first track of this demographic trend was the prosperous London haberdasher, who could also reasonably claim to be the first epidemiologist. John Graunt was described by polymath John Aubrey, author of *Brief Lives*, as 'a pleasant facetious [waggish] companion and very hospitable'. Graunt's analytical book *Natural and Political Observations Made upon the Bills of Mortality* published in 1662 greatly impressed Charles II and won its author election to the Royal Society, although having little effect on the plague of 1665–67. Unfortunately he lost his grand house in the Great Fire and afterwards went bankrupt, dying of liver disease at the age of 53.

Across the Channel in France, the north of the country was at first spared the worst ravages of the plague due to rigorous measures ordained by the parliaments of Rouen and Paris. Yet, as the plague died down in England, it went from strength to strength in France, reaching Lille and Cambrai by the end of 1667 and by summer of 1668 Amiens, Beauvais, Reims, Le Havre and Dieppe. Louis XIV's chief minister J-P. Colbert (1619–1683)[7] saved the capital by a *cordon sanitaire* rigorously imposed around its northern suburbs and ensured observance of his isolation rules by teams of deputies, who overruled all complaints that they were killing commerce. This same conflict of economic arguments against good medical practice would reappear in the Covid-19 pandemic of 2019–20.

By spring of 1670 the plague in France was all but ended.[8] Why did the Great Plague gradually die out? At the time, theories ranged from coincident astronomical influences to better nutrition to a new fashion of using soap for the body and in washing clothes, and taking off one's day clothes on going to bed – thus making infestation by insect parasites more difficult – to the reorientation of commerce with the New World, to the simple fact that survivors had acquired immunity to the as yet unknown bacterium later dubbed *Y. pestis*.

Chapter 9

The Great Fire

Long before the Great Fire of 1666, London had burned many times at irregular intervals, as had every large town in England, due to the closeness of the houses, their jettied upper storeys nearly touching those opposite and the flammable materials of which they were made. The thatched roofs were a particular fire hazard.

In the middle of the first century of the Common Era, after the death of Prasutagas, chief of the Iceni, the territory of that tribe should have passed jointly to the Roman emperor and Prasutagas' widow Boudicca under the terms of the Iceni's treaty of alliance with Rome. Instead, Rome claimed it all. For disputing this, Boudicca was publicly flogged and her daughters gang-raped by legionaries. In revenge, she launched a rebellion with an army of her own people and British allies, first sacking Camulodunum, modern Colchester. Marching her army on to Londinium, they burned the town down, the violence of the conflagration being so great that some coins of the time have been excavated from the mud of the Thames melted together into a solid mass. Verulamium – the modern St Albans – was also put to the sack and burned.

Londinium was rebuilt, but in 122 CE a mysterious fire destroyed much of the re-building. In the Anglo-Saxon period several more fires caused great damage. In 675 a fire destroyed much of the city including the first, wooden, St Paul's cathedral. More fires happened in 764, 798, 852, 893. The re-built St Paul's was destroyed again in the fire of 982. After the Norman Conquest, London burned again in 1077 and 1087, when it was said that the greater part of the city was destroyed, including, for the third time, St Paul's. In 1135 another extensive fire in the city was attributed to thatched roofs carrying the flames from one building to the next across the very narrow streets. A major casualty was the dilapidated wooden London bridge and the buildings on it, through which the fire flashed from one bank to the other, burning down homes and commercial property for 1.5 miles along the banks of the river.

In 1189 a city ordinance known as the Assize of Buildings – an early form of building regulations – required for this reason that thatch be no longer used in roofing. The problem was that many city-dwellers could not afford any other form of roofing material. Thus the requirement was more honoured in the breach than the observance, as reflected by the requirement that each alderman should equip himself with a long and stout iron hook, to pull burning thatch down to ground level, where it could be doused with water. To make this possible, householders were required to keep sturdy ladders on the premises and to maintain a full barrel of water in the dry summer months. Of course, many did not comply. The bridge was rebuilt in stone but, to raise revenue, King John allowed timber-framed houses to be built along it. When a fire started in Southwark and flashed through the houses across London bridge, hundreds of people were burned to death, but the masonry structure of the bridge was left more or less intact.

After this fire, owners of houses with thatched roofs were given just a week to get rid of them, or have them torn down by the aldermen. In defiance of the new roofing regulations, some houses continued to be thatched and in 1377 an enquiry by the alderman of Colmanstrete ward heard evidence that houses belonging to six citizens and the *hoggesty* of a seventh were still thatched. The offenders were given forty days to strip the thatch under threat of having it done by the sheriffs and paying a fine of 40 shillings. Even so, five years later, there were still fifteen thatched houses in Chancery Lane.

In addition, throughout the Middle Ages, tons of flammable hay and straw were brought into the city each day to feed the hundreds of animals stabled there. Milk was a very profitable commodity, selling at 2¼ pence a pint, but it had to be fresh and the only way to ensure that was to walk the cow to the customer's house and milk it there directly into the householder's pot. At the time, the borough of Hackney alone was home to 600 cows, as well as horses and other domestic animals. Not only were these animals susceptible to human diseases, but all the resultant dung rendered large parts of the city insanitary.

In 1633 another fire in the houses along the bridge destroyed forty-two buildings and spread along the north bank for half a mile, which may have been a good thing because the damage constituted a fire-break that prevented the Great Fire of 1666 from crossing the river. Ironically, the Great Fire of London began, not in a thatched house, stable or *hoggesty*, but in the early hours of 2 September in the basement of a bakery with tiled roof in Pudding Lane owned by the king's baker Thomas Farrinor. He swore afterward that the fire had been raked out when he retired to bed at 10 p.m., but smouldering embers ignited some kindling stacked nearby. About 2 a.m. the family awoke, choking from the smoke, and found flames coming up the stairs. To escape the flames, Farrinor climbed through an upstairs window with his wife, son, daughter and a servant. The maid panicked. Overcome by flames or smoke, she became the fire's first victim. Although an estimated 80,000 Londoners lost their homes and businesses that night and in the following days, there are believed to have been only a handful of other fatalities.

At the end of a long summer drought, the neighbouring timber-framed buildings rapidly caught fire, their timbers being weather-proofed with pitch. The typical six- or seven-storey timbered London tenement houses had projecting upper floors, which all but met those of the houses opposite. In 1661 Charles II had ruled against this style of building as a fire risk, but the landlords' greed and the corruption of the magistrates had undone all the good he intended. In 1665 he again warned of the fire danger, backing up the warning with the threat of imprisonment for contraventions and the demolition of offending buildings. This too had little effect.

Thus the fire leaped across Fish Street Hill, engulfing the Star Inn. Driven by a strong northeast wind, it spread rapidly into Thames Street, igniting all the flammable goods in the river-front warehouses such as pitch, tallow and oil, against which the primitive firefighting means of men passing to each other wooden buckets of water; was useless. One or two primitive mobile pumps were available, but whether they were used is unknown . The normal way to halt a major fire was to demolish houses in the fire's path, to prevent its spread but Lord Mayor Thomas Bloodworth hesitated to give the order in case he was held liable for the cost of rebuilding. On Sunday 2 September 1666 Pepys' diary entry was:

> Jane called us up about three in the morning, to tell us of a great fire they saw in the City. So I rose and slipped on my nightgowne, and went to her window, and thought it to be on the backside of Marke-lane at the farthest; but, being unused to such fires as followed, I thought it far enough off; and so went to bed again and to sleep. About seven rose

again to dress myself, and there looked out at the window, and saw the fire not so much as it was and further off. So to my closett to set things to rights after yesterday's cleaning.

By and by Jane comes and tells me that she hears that above 300 houses have been burned down to-night by the fire we saw, and that it is now burning down all Fish-street, by London Bridge. So I made myself ready presently, and walked to the Tower, and there got up upon one of the high places, Sir J. Robinson's little son going up with me; and there I did see the houses at that end of the bridge all on fire, and an infinite great fire on this and the other side the end of the bridge; which, among other people, did trouble me for poor little Michell and our Sarah on the bridge. So down, with my heart full of trouble, to the Lieutenant of the Tower, who tells me that it begun this morning in the King's baker's house in Pudding-lane, and that it hath burned St. Magnus's Church and most part of Fish-street already. So I down to the water-side, and there got a boat and through bridge, and there saw a lamentable fire.

Ever since King Charles I's fatal attempt to secure absolute power, the royal army was not welcome in the predominantly pro-parliament city, which explains why soldiers were not already fighting the fire. Several hundred night watchmen usually patrolled the streets of the city at night, and would normally have raised the 'trained bands' or local militia, who did have some fire-fighting equipment, but nowhere near enough. Their primitive pumps required a supply of water by connection to one of the few water mains or access to the river, where unfortunately, several pumps fell into the water and were lost. Soon, the pressure in the buried elmwood water mains failed entirely after flames destroyed the huge water wheels moored under London bridge, which pumped water up to the water tower in Cornhill.

On 4 September John Evelyn took a coach from Deptford to Southwark, in order to view the conflagration across the river from the left bank of the Thames. He commented that people were too dazed to fight the fire as it approached their houses. Evelyn likened the scene of destruction to the sack of Troy by the Greeks. It seemed to him that the city of London could never be rebuilt. The easterly wind must have changed direction, because the flames were advancing northward by mid-afternoon, reaching Lombard Street and Cheapside and heading for the smart shops of Cornhill. Evelyn commented that the very stones of houses were exploding with the heat; in the streets ran rivers of boiling lead from the roofs and gutters. It seemed that everyone in London was panicking. The 18-foot-high Roman wall enclosing the city had only eight congested gates by which to leave, these being soon jammed by distraught people trying to get out with their bundles, carts, horses, and wagons. Once the fire had spread along the north bank of the Thames, escape by water would be impossible. Evelyn had a particular care on September 5 for the 'many wounded and sick men' he had in St Bartholomew's Hospital and the Savoy, directly in the path of the fire, but the wind changed again, and they were saved.

When the flames eventually died down, the Great Fire of London had destroyed no less than 13,200 houses, three city gates, the entire Royal Exchange building, and fifty-two livery company halls, together with law courts, gaols and so many official buildings that the administration of the city ground to a halt. Eighty-seven churches, were destroyed, including St Paul's Cathedral, which enabled Sir Christopher Wren to build his masterpiece as replacement. Six months later, Pepys reported some smoke still emerging from cellars, where stuff had been smouldering all that time beneath the rubble. He himself was so traumatised by living through the fire that he could not sleep at night, for fear of it somehow re-kindling itself and killing him in his slumbers.

It was said afterward that the Great Fire must have killed off all the rats and fleas, thus stopping the epidemic. With hindsight, however, the fire had little effect on the plague, which was already dying down beforehand and some people continued to die of it well into the 1670s. The Rebuilding Act of February 1667, pushed through by King Charles II and his brother James, Duke of York, was praised by many, including Samuel Pepys, as a far-sighted, although somewhat draconian, measure against fires in the city. The exterior walls of all new buildings had to be constructed of brick or stone – not just for the looks, but because experience in other countries found the masonry-built houses of the rich provided far more security against entry of rats and their fleas than the wood-framed lath and plaster walls of the poor. This may have explained the lesser mortality of the affluent parishes. In addition, a maximum number of storeys per house was imposed for a fixed number of dwellings, lessening intra-mural crowding. Many timber-framed houses were torn down and pavements created, to give more separation. The medieval system of guilds was re-formed and an appeal was made for 'all carpenters, bricklayers, masons, plasterers & joiners' to help with reconstruction.[2] The requirement for 'outsides of all Buildings in and about the said Citty to henceforth be made of Bricke or Stone' was not simply an anti-plague and anti-fire measure, but also because of the government's need for timber to build ships. Six decades earlier King James I of England had also required new houses in London to be made of masonry for this reason. Repeated royal proclamations sometimes mentioned that these houses would be fire-resistant, but the aim was to keep the mature oak of the English forests for the navy-yards.

Most readers familiar with the modern Mediterranean landscape are unaware that 2,000 years ago the inland sea was surrounded with mature oak forests that were cut down to make tens of thousands of ships, both merchant vessels and naval galleys. The amount of timber in all those 'wooden walls' was astronomical and such was the requirement for structural timbers of a particular shape that several dozen huge trees would be felled before all the required timber for one ship was obtained. Britain's oak forests suffered similarly. In the Mediterranean, of course, any re-planting of oak was rendered useless by the extensive pasturing of goats, whose tendency to eat everything had earned them the title 'fathers of the desert'.

In the aftermath of the Rebuilding Act, London's masonry exterior walls may have looked good and made intrusion by rats harder, but all the interior walls and ceilings of ordinary homes were still made of lath and plaster. The floors were wooden and tiled roofs were heavy, requiring stout load-bearing beams, rafters, trusses, battens and purlins – so much wood in fact that a fire starting inside a dwelling would find plenty of combustible material above it, no matter what the exterior walls were made of.

The London School of Economics analysis of the plague's spreading is based on records of roughly 930,000 burials and 630,000 baptisms to reconstruct the patterns of birth and death in London from 1560 to 1665. Although not complete, the Bills of Mortality consulted cover the ninety-seven parishes within the walls; the sixteen parishes outside the walls, twelve parishes in Middlesex and Surrey and the five parishes of Westminster. Not belonging to any parish were the Inns of Court and the

Tower of London. Between 1560 and 1600 the population of London doubled, with all the living standards, sanitation and other stresses which that implies. Economically, whereas the Black Death of the fourteenth century led to important rises in living standards, it is notable that later plague mortality had little impact on wages because new migrants rapidly replaced dead Londoners.

This analysis gives the lie to the theory that plagues arrived each time aboard ships engaged in international commerce because London's docks were in the east, whereas plagues started in the poor northern suburban parishes. Also, if plagues spread each time into Northern Europe from the Mediterranean, one would expect each outbreak to begin in Italy, followed by Spain and France, with the Low Countries and Britain afterwards. This is not the case. Work by E.A. Wrigley and R.S. Schofield found that mortality peaked in March and reached a minimum in July.[3] Yet plague deaths peaked in the autumn. Typhus, however, shows little seasonality apart from a tendency to virulence in the colder season.

Restoration theatre proved a ladder for some women to rise high in society, female parts previously having been played in skirts by boys or slender men. Charles II had many mistresses, who flaunted their standing at court. Queen Catherine being unable to keep a pregnancy to full term and provide an heir to the throne, came to accept this state of affairs. Evelyn's venom was aimed at, among other actresses, Mrs Davenport, who played Roxolana, and was 'my Lord Oxford's Miss'; Mrs Uphill was Sir R. Howard's temptress; and Mrs Hughes ensnared Prince Rupert. The women's titles did not indicate marital status, but merely that they were aged twenty-one or older.

The most enduringly famous of these liberated ladies was Nell Gwynne, adored by Pepys, who called her 'pretty, witty Nell' and considered her a wonderful actress. She later caught Charles II's eye. Since her two earlier long-term lovers were Charles Hart, an actor, and Charles Sackville, 6th Earl of Dorset, she took to calling the king 'Charles the Third'. She bore him two sons named Charles and James Beauclerk in their sixteen-year relationship. On a visit to her dwelling by the king, she called her son Charles to her: 'Come here, you little bastard, and meet your father.' The king protested, to which she replied, 'You have given me no other label by which to call him.' Her ploy worked. Charles II ennobled the boy, making him Duke of St Albans.

Divine justice did not strike down these loose women. On the contrary, on 28 October Evelyn commented that the pestilence in Deptford was abating 'through God's mercy'. Life, it seemed was back to normal, the only sign of the infection the large numbers of plague pits spread all over London within and outside the walls. When full and covered up, the ground above each pit was liberally dosed with vinegar used as a disinfectant. Many of London's green spaces, where people today walk their dogs, exercise or play games, are above plague pits. By Aldgate Underground station was a pit described by Daniel Defoe in his book *A Journal of the Plague Year*:

> A terrible pit it was, and I could not resist my curiosity to go and see it. As near as I may judge, it was about forty feet in length, and about fifteen or sixteen feet broad, and at the time I first looked at it, about nine feet deep; but it was said they dug it near twenty feet deep afterwards in one part of it, till they could go no deeper for the water; for they had, it seems, dug several large pits before this. For though the plague was long a-coming to our parish, yet, when it did come, there was no parish in or about London where it raged with such violence as in the two parishes of Aldgate and Whitechappel.

Also noted by Defoe in his book was Hand Alley in Bishopsgate – now renamed New Street. At the time a green field, it was dug up and used to bury the victims of Bishopsgate and many others. Golden Square in Soho was another pit, described by Lord Macaulay in 1685:

> A field not to be passed without a shudder by any Londoner of that age. There, as in a place far from the haunts of men, had been dug, twenty years before, when the great plague was raging, a pit into which the dead carts had nightly shot corpses by scores.

It was popularly believed that the earth was deeply tainted with infection, and could not be disturbed without imminent risk to human life. The largest pit in London was the one unearthed by the Crossrail workers in March 2013 in Charterhouse Square, Farringdon, where the remains of 50,000 plague victims are believed to lie. South of the Thames, in Southwark, the Cross Bones graveyard was an unconsecrated burial ground where thousands of prostitutes were interred, and which was pressed into service in 1665 as a plague pit overseen by the churchwardens of St Saviour's parish. At the depot on the southern end of the Bakerloo Line is a runaway line for trains unable to stop. Any passengers on such trains may not know that this tunnel runs right through a plague pit, from which they are separated just by the brick-lined tunnel walls. As its name suggests, Pitfield Street in Hoxton was used as a large plague pit.

Users of neighbouring Shoreditch Park requested to *Keep off the Grass* may not know what lies below! Hounsditch in the City owes its name to its function during the Roman occupation of Britain (43–410 CE) as a place to dispose of dead dogs. There are several plague pits here, where, twelve and a half centuries later, human corpses 'went to the dogs'. Armour House at the junction of St Martins LeGrand and Gresham St was built with a sub-basement bridging a plague pit. It is locally believed that several building applications have been rejected for the triangular green space called Shepherd's Bush Common for fear of disturbing the plague pit under the grass. Vincent Square in Westminster is a thirteen-acre green space owned by Westminster School, some of whose playing fields here are located above the large plague pit then called Tothill Fields.[5]

Chapter 10

Plague, Typhus, Cholera
Take Your Pick

The Great Plague of London was over, but lesser outbreaks continued the grisly work elsewhere in England for some years. Meanwhile, the capital had its shares of problems caused by the plague. Defoe comments on the widespread unemployment caused by the collapse of the economy, leading the upper classes to fear, as he put it:

> that Desperation should push the People upon Tumults. And cause them to rifle the houses of rich Men who had fled London, and plunder the Markets of Provisions; in which case the Country People, who brought Provisions very freely and boldly to Town, would ha' been terrified from coming any more, and the Town would ha' sunk under an unavoidable Famine.
>
> But the Prudence of my Lord Mayor, and the Court of Aldermen within the City, and of the Justices of the Peace in the Outparts [ensured] ... that the poor People were kept quiet and their Wants everywhere relieved, as far as was possible to be done ...

by distributing the funds provided as charity for the purpose and finding work for the unemployed. With 10,000 houses shut up, a day watchman and a night watchman were required for each one. This, as Defore puts it, 'gave opportunity to employ a great Number of poor Men'. Unemployed women were similarly employed as 'Nurses to tend the Sick in all Places.'[1] Defoe also commented that, although the Bills of Mortality totalled those dead of the plague in London at 68,590, a truer figure would have been 100,000, if all those not counted for various reasons had been included.

In many other places, plague deaths continued. In 1708 the army of Swedish King Charles XII was forced to retreat after a previously successful campaign in southern Russia when its numbers were significantly reduced by plague. In 1720 the ship *Grand Saint Antoine* coming from the Middle East arrived in the French Mediterranean port of Marseille. The vessel was officially quarantined, but the shipowner was the deputy mayor of the city and forced the premature unloading of its cargo so that he could realise his investment sooner. Rats came ashore with the cargo, their infected fleas rapidly spreading across the city, sparking an epidemic. People died by the thousands, the piles of bodies dumped in the streets growing so large that convict labourers had to be conscripted to remove and bury the corpses in plague pits. Outside the city, plague walls were hurriedly built, but failed to contain the pestilence, which killed some 100,000 people in southern France before dying out in 1722.

In November 1741 Prague was surrendered to the French after 30,000 Austrian defenders died of plague. Some historians even thought that the French Revolution was decided in 1792 by an attack of dysentery that reduced the armies of Prussia and Austria from 42,000 men to less than 30,000, forcing them to retreat back across the Rhine. In 1801 Haiti, across the Atlantic, was invaded by Napoleon's General Leclerc to put down the rebellion of Toussaint L'Ouverture. Of Leclerc's 25,000 force only 3,000 survived an attack of yellow fever, and had to be evacuated, leaving Haiti free of French domination.[2]

Half a century later, the Crimean war, famous for the suicidal charge of the Light Brigade, was also a marvellous opportunity for epidemics. In December 1854 and December of 1855 two separate outbreaks of lice-borne typhus raged in the Russian forces. Lice also affected the British and French invaders while still travelling on their transport ships to Constantinople and Turkey, before they even landed on the peninsula. After the battle of the Alma on 20 September 1854, cholera brought by the British troops turned into an epidemic that afflicted all the Allied armies – British, French, Turkish and Egyptian – and crossed the lines to hit the Russian defenders also. When the figures were added up, twice as many Allied soldiers died of disease as from wounds: 67,040 as against 25,303. In the Russian lines roughly the same number died from wounds as from disease: 38,000 in each case. The *modus operandi* of this killer disease is devastatingly simple: nausea, vomiting and continuous diarrhoea that dehydrates the body at the rate of a litre every hour until death quickly ensues.

It was simply accepted by the army medics as inevitable until an extraordinary 34-year-old woman arrived from England. Florence Nightingale was born on 12 May 1820 into a wealthy British family then living in Florence, which is how she got the name. After the family moved back to England in 1821, her father having advanced ideas about girls' education, both Florence and her sister were tutored in history, mathematics, Italian, classical literature and philosophy. Growing up, Florence at first respected her mother's and sister's views that a women of her class should settle down to marriage and childbearing after an early marriage. With an annual income settled on her by her father of £500 – worth £40,000 in today's money– she had no need to work, but during a tour of Egypt in 1850 she experienced what may be called a religious experience, and decided to devote her life to the service of humanity by fighting disease. The first step was to spend four months in a German Lutheran religious community, where Pastor Theodor Flieder tended the sick and poor with a staff of deaconesses acting as his nurses. On returning to London, Florence took the post of matron (August 1853–October 1854) of the Institute for the Care of Sick Gentlewomen.

The Crimean war broke out in October 1853, lasting until February 1856, pitting the coalition of English, French, Turkish and Egyptian forces against the Tsarist Russian garrison of the peninsula. The avowed aim of the coalition was to prevent the Russian Black Sea Fleet forcing a passage through the Bosphorus and emerging in the Mediterranean. However, the Allies' incompetent generals – British C-in-C Lord Raglan was so confused that he thought he was still fighting what he called 'those Frenchies' in Spain – caused hundreds of thousands of deaths from malnutrition and frostbite in summer uniforms when soldiers' tents blew away in winter blizzards, as just one example. As with all armies on campaign previously, more casualties were lost to disease and gangrene than in combat. When the critical reports of *Times* correspondent William Russell reached London, telling of the appalling conditions in the main military hospital in Scutari (modern Üsküdar) across the Bosphorus from Constantinople, Florence decided that her moment had come. She recruited a team of thirty-eight volunteer nurses and fifteen nuns, instructing them in her method of nursing – a mixture of intelligence and hygiene, arriving in Turkey in October 1854, to find that not only were they refused permission to travel to the peninsula where the fighting was going on, they were also not welcome in the main base hospital at Üsküdar, the army doctors at first refusing them entry to the wards. Only when they were overwhelmed by a massive influx of wounded after the battle of Inkerman, did the medics reluctantly admit Florence and her nurses.

She found men dying of typhoid, typhus, cholera and dysentery in filthy wards where even the sewage system did not work. She first requisitioned 200 scrubbing brushes and a vast quantity of carbolic soap, with which the nurses had to scrub down floors, walls and ceilings of the wards allocated to her, which were infested with rats and fleas. She also set up a laundry, where the wounded men's filthy and verminous clothing could be washed, and a proper kitchen to cook them nourishing meals. The first requirement of her nursing was washing hands between patients – a measure that would have saved so many women's lives in the lying-in hospitals of Paris and London a century later. The death rate in the hospital had been 44 per cent before her arrival; she brought it down to 2.2 per cent by imposing her rules of hygiene.[3] A gifted mathematician, Florence also displayed great ability for collecting, analysing and presenting data, which earned her the respect of modern epidemiologists. Although she did not invent the pie chart, her polar charts recording needless fatalities in the Crimean war popularised this means of presenting information.

Cholera, perhaps the greatest scourge in the Crimea, is an interesting disease, of which the first recorded outbreak was in 1817 in the river deltas near Calcutta, where it still thrives. It found a 'home from home' on the other side of the world, killing half a million people in New York in 1832 and travelled on to infect Central and South America widely in 1868. Since then, cholera has caused seven epidemics, of which the first six were all probably due to the original bacillus, designated *type 01* with the last caused by a mutant form designated *El Tor*. There is also a newcomer to the collection of lethal diseases given the identity of *type 0139* at the cholera research institution in Vellore.

Although cholera only occurs now in Britain among recent immigrants, there was a famous outbreak in 1854 in Soho, west central London. Fortunately for London, Dr John Snow (1813–1858) had worked with a colleague in Newcastle on previous outbreaks in England. He was an exceptional doctor and anesthesiologist working at Westminster

Hospital, with an interest in public health, now remembered as a pioneer epidemiologist and a founder member of the Epidemiological Society of London, formed just four years before the outbreak.

Rightly disbelieving the medieval theory of miasmas, Snow approached the Soho outbreak logically, by talking to residents of the affected area, where 600 people had recently died. He plotted the whereabouts of each affected household by marking dots on a large-scale map and concluded that the common cause was a widely used public water pump in Broad Street, Soho – now Broadwick Street – which proved to have been dug only three feet from a disused cesspool swarming with the flagellate bacillus *vibrio cholerae* pathogen, which leaked into the well. With his available microscopes, he could not detect *cryptosporidium*, the source of the cholera, but wrote matter-of-factly to the editor of the *Medical Times and Gazette*:

> I had an interview with the Board of Guardians of St James's parish, on the evening of [7 September], and represented [my findings] to them. In consequence of what I said, the handle of the pump was removed on the following day.

End of outbreak. Snow went on to demonstrate statistically that people in homes using water from the Southwark and Vauxhall water company, which drew its supply from sewage-polluted stretches of the Thames, had fourteen times more chance of getting cholera than customers of the Lambeth water company, which drew its supplies from the unpolluted Seething Wells up-river. Impressed, Benjamin Disraeli and other members of parliament took up the cause of clean water and hygienic sewage disposal against the vested interest of landlords and the water companies

Sadly, in many regions of the Third World where middle-class and rich people drink only bottled mineral water, the poor continue to drink water from the rivers into which raw sewage is dumped up-stream. Chlorination, which could save countless lives, is not practised even in Lima, the capital of Peru, the alibi of the responsible officials being that chlorine is carcinogenic. The real reason is bureaucratic corruption, which ensures that poor Peruvians continue to die from cholera despite the fact that modern sanitation and sewage disposal would eliminate it. Even for people who now contract it, there is since 1968, a simple cure. A mixture of equal proportions of glucose and salts is given to the sufferer; the glucose enables the salts to pass through the intestinal wall and replace lost body fluids and vital salts. This reduces mortality from 50 per cent to less than 1 per cent. Yet WHO estimates that cholera continues to kill 143,000 people a year in the Third World.

Another disease spread by contamination of drinking water is typhoid, caused by *salmonella typhii*, not to be confused with *salmonella enterica*. Typhoid's most famous casualty among the 50,000 British victims of the 1861 epidemic was Prince Albert, the German consort of Queen Victoria. This was a difficult disease to eradicate because even cured sufferers still had the bacilli in their bodies and excreted them alive, launching a new round of infection. Usually the bacilli gradually reduce in number, but in some cases they do not and the former sufferers become enduring vectors for the disease. The most famous case was Mary Mallon, an Irish cook working in New York who infected every family for whom she worked, earning the nickname Typhoid Mary. Changing jobs frequently, and infecting each family that employed her, she was finally tracked down in 1906 by George Soper, a major in the US Army Sanitary Corps. After she escaped from preventive detention, imposed to prevent her infecting ever more employers and their families, she returned to kitchen work under different names and continued to infect people, sometimes fatally, and even the nurses in a hospital that employed her. The only way of preventing her lethal life of freedom was a return to compulsory solitary incarceration, which ended when she died in 1938.

Typhus is caused by different bacteria – *rickettsia typhii* in the case of endemic typhus, also known as murine typhus or jail fever, whereas *rickettsia prowazekii* is the usual bacterial cause of epidemic typhus. This can, if untreated, kill up to 60 per cent of those infected. Although long thought to be viruses because they are so small, these bacteria are now controlled with antibiotics. Mankind's great enemies in this area are the head and body lice afflicting humans since time immemorial, respectively designated *pediculus humanus capitis* and *pediculus humanus corporis*. Both species ran amok in wars, where the men lacked water for washing and wore the same clothes day and night for weeks on end. In the trench warfare of the First World War, lice were ubiquitous, as they had been in the Crimea. In the infamous Nazi concentration and extermination camps during the Second World War notices in the grossly overcrowded and insanitary barracks bore the warning *Ein Laus = der Tod* – one louse and you die. Himmler's murderous camp staff and their underlings were not worried about infected prisoners dying, but were terrified that the prisoners' lice might transfer to their guards and infect them with typhus.

The symptoms, not all of which may be present in each sufferer, include abdominal and back pain, headaches, joint and muscle pain, a hacking dry cough, nausea and vomiting, fever up to 41.1 degrees Centigrade(106 degrees Fahrenheit), a red rash spreading all over the body, confusion, low blood pressure and sensitivity to bright lights. With all that armoury at the disposal of typhus, death of the sufferers in Himmler's camps may have come as a blessed release.

Technically speaking, typhus is an infection by rickettsial bacteria from the bite of an arthropod parasite such as an infected flea, louse, tick or mite, each species specialising in one type of typhus. The bite itches, causing the sufferer to scratch it and spread the infection, probably by letting the arthropod's minute excreta cross the skin barrier through tiny scratches. In endemic or murine typhus the symptoms last a couple of weeks, but are less severe.

A third type of typhus is known as scrub typhus. In addition to all the symptoms above, this produces swollen lymph nodes and exhaustion, but is generally restricted to South American and African countries with widespread poverty, poor sanitation and cramped living conditions. As though all that is not enough, untreated typhus may lead to hepatitis, hypovolaemia and bleeding in the intestines.

In the nineteenth century, people of all classes had to be aware of the risks. Sir Moses Montefiore (1784–1885) was an Italian-born Victorian banker, philanthropist, knight of the realm and sheriff of London, who rose from poverty to great wealth. After retiring from business, in 1831 he purchased Eastcliffe Lodge, a mock-Gothic mansion set in a country estate outside the then-fashionable seaside resort of Ramsgate which had formerly been owned by a brother of the Duke of Wellington. On Sir Moses' eighty-ninth birthday a local paper, instead of congratulating him, mistakenly ran his obituary. The very much alive banker foreshadowed Mark Twain's later comment on a similar mistake by writing to the editor: 'I thank God to have been able to hear of the rumour, and to read an account of the same with my own eyes, without using spectacles.' With the same sense of humour, when seated at a dinner party next to an anti-Semitic English nobleman who remarked that he was recently returned from a trip to Japan where, he said 'there were neither pigs nor Jews,' Montefiore responded, 'In that case both you and I should go there, so they have a sample of each.'

Quick wit is amusing, but Sir Moses also had connections at the highest level, which enabled him to combine with the English branch of the international Rothschild bankers to raise a loan enabling the British government to compensate plantation owners under the Slavery Abolition Act of 1833, which abolished slavery in the British Empire. But his main philanthropic activities were aiding persecuted Jews in several countries by personally pleading with, and presumably appropriately rewarding, the Ottoman sultan, the pope, the tsar of Russia, and other heads of state.

Yet Montefiore's elevated social status, privileges and huge wealth were no protection against disease in the nineteenth century. Travelling several times to Turkish-occupied Palestine, to oversee his good works there, he financed some of the first *kibbutzim* and invested in alms houses, still to be seen in Jerusalem. He also paid for agricultural training for poor Jews and provided funds to improve their inadequate diet. Under Turkish law, it was illegal to sell land to Jews and other would-be purchasers who were not Muslims. As a protective measure, Montefiore also paid for censuses of his co-religionists in 1839, 1849, 1855, 1866 and 1875 earning him the honorific Hebrew title of *ha-Sar* or the Prince.

If life in Palestine was difficult, simply getting there was not easy even for one of the most powerful and rich men in Europe. The eastern Mediterranean was still haunted by pirates eager to take hostage a traveller whose ransom would be very high, cholera was widespread and malarial mosquitoes common. Not until July 1897, after two years of research, did an unconventional British army medical officer Ronald Ross (1857–1932), when dissecting a female anopheles mosquito under the microscope, find falciparum parasites in the stomach and prove the connection between these mosquitoes carrying the malaria pathogen and their human victims by injecting it in their blood-thinning saliva. He also developed mathematical models of malaria transmission and, in 1902, was awarded a Nobel Prize for his work.

The Montefiores were travelling across Europe in 1839 in their private enclosed carriage, changing horses regularly, and availing themselves of the luxuries of riverboat paddle steamers when available. Comfort was important; on one visit to Palestine, the round trip took them ten months. Reaching the Mediterranean outbound, they boarded a ship for Malta, an important international transit port in the Victorian age. On arrival, passengers and cargo transferred to different ships for their onward journey. Two years later Thomas Cook invented modern tour-group travel but the Montefores had to land in Valetta harbour and wait for a suitable vessel to take them further, negotiating with its captain the price for their onward journey.

Malta was then controlled by the Ottoman Sultanate, which operated a sophisticated quarantine *lazaretto*[4] on Manoel Island for any well-heeled passengers. This luxury hotel had been upgraded the previous year by the governor of Malta, and could accommodate several dozen people in capacious suites, securely separated and distanced from each other so no infection would be transmitted while they waited out their quarantine period after medical examination of their skin, the inside the mouth and elsewhere. For passengers' baggage there were compulsory customs inspection and fumigation facilities. Travellers coming from an area known to have cholera or other infectious diseases had to stay in isolated confinement for a set period, sometimes of several weeks.

The news from Palestine was not good: there was plague in Jerusalem and at the port-city of Jaffa, where they had intended to land. Sir Moses wanted to send home his wife and most of their large entourage, to reduce their risk of exposure to plague. Well aware of the risks – on one trip her diary mentioned quarantine thirty-eight times – Lady Judith insisted on continuing the journey, armed with a certificate of good health from the *lazaretto*. On 3 May 1839 Montefiore's party was ferried out to the SS *Megara,* accompanied by a quarantine boat to ensure there was no contact with any vessel or person that had not been quarantined. The *Megara* was bound for Alexandria in Egypt to land some passengers and pick up others, load some freight and allow passengers to collect mail and send letters home and to their destinations by faster, smaller ships. Before any of this could be done, the captain had to show the Maltese health certificates to the Egyptian authorities. To avoid personal contact, he was required to hand them over with a pair of tongs.

The passengers aboard the *Megara* were disturbed by the hostilities between the Ottoman sultan and Mehmet Ali, the pasha of Egypt, who also ruled Palestine and Syria. Wishing to proceed as soon as possible, the Montefiores learned that Jaffa – the nearest port to Jeruslem – was closed because of the plague, so they would have to sail past it and land at Beirut in modern Lebanon. From there, after more quarantine formalities, they hoped to complete their journey by riding on horseback for 250 miles across the Galilean and Judean mountains. In addition to plague and cholera, the risks of robbery or murder by local brigands obliged them to hire a squad of armed soldiers for protection. The Beirut *lazaretto* was a far cry from the luxury of Malta. From the window of Lady Judith's uncomfortable bedroom rows of graves were visible, where plague victims had hastily been buried. In the ill-lit corridor just outside her door a large poisonous snake was killed. While she kept to her bed for several days, possibly with food poisoning, letters were received from Sir Moses' contacts in Jerusalem, all having been cooked in ovens on arrival in Beirut to kill any plague bacteria.

Quarantine over, he and his young wife were allowed to visit friends' homes before departing in their armed convoy, heading for the ancient Galilean cities of Safed and Tiberias on Lake Galilee, regularly changing their route to avoid villages with plague and/or cholera. While travelling, the Montefiores slept on a bed in a tent, but most of their companions had to sleep on the ground under the stars, risking the bites of disease-carrying ticks and sand-flies. Ibrahim, the cook, had to both procure the food from local sources and prepare it. In the day-time, Lady Judith rode side-saddle, as most Victorian ladies did, but wore a pistol for her personal defence. At Nablus in Samaria they were not allowed to sleep in the town, in case they brought plague with them, but were obliged to camp outside the walls, protected by their soldiers. Foreshadowing the contradictions of Covid-19 precautions in Britain, they were, however, allowed to go into the town during daylight, for sightseeing and to consult Sir Moses' contacts there.

Some weeks after leaving Beirut, the party reached Jerusalem. The daily death toll from cholera was high, so they camped outside on *har ha-zetim* – the Mount of Olives – for safety from disease, if not from robbers. News of their arrival brought visitors across the valley of the Kidron stream, begging for assistance. Written petitions had to be left on the ground and picked up with tongs, to avoid person-to-person contact. The British consul also visited these important visitors, telling them that many Jews in the city were so poor they had to eat grass and weeds, and attributing to this the virulence of the plague and cholera. The Muslim governor of Jerusalem also came, inviting Sir Moses and Lady Judith to enjoy a magnificent ceremonial reception in the city, but they refused, for fear of infection. In their guarded camp on the Mount of Olives, they did at least accept gifts of wine and food, including five live sheep, which Ibrahim slaughtered one by one, and cooked.

It being difficult to reject Arab hospitality without causing grave offence, eventually Sir Moses and Lady Judith consented to enter the city on fine Arab mounts, loaned to them for the occasion, and escorted by an imposing mounted guard of honour. They were welcomed by the whole Jewish population of the city, who pressed in on them so tightly that their bodyguard was overcome and all hope of social distancing abandoned, as happened also when they moved on to Hebron. By then, their sacks formerly filled with gold coins were empty and an urgent message was sent to a bank in Beirut for more, which had to be transported by another armed convoy. Hoping to take ship at Jaffa, they were refused entry because of the plague still rampant there, but bribed the quarantine superintendent to give them a clean bill of health and rode and camped their way northwards along the coast back to Beirut. Even this was not so easy. Arriving at Mount Carmel, not intending to stay long in Haifa, they were informed that they must fulfil a 2-week quarantine in a cordoned-off area despite the health certificate from Jaffa. Bribery and a visit from the British consul had this modified on condition they immersed themselves, their entourage, their horses, mules, bedding and tents in the sea – to 'sterilise' everything.

Finally heaving sighs of relief, they boarded a ship in Beirut, bound for Alexandria. So far, so good. But on arrival in Malta they were quarantined in strict isolation again in the *lazaretto*. Such was the reality of travel, even for the ultra-rich, in the 1840s. Undeterred, Sir Moses made a total of six trips to Palestine, the last in 1874 when he was ninety years old.

The quarantine stations in the Mediterranean continued to function until 1936, nearly twenty years after the Spanish Flu pandemic. Is this how long some of the COVID-19 crisis restrictions will last?

Chapter 11

Getting to Know the Enemy

In 1855 a rebellion erupted in China's Yunnan province. Imperial troops sent from Beijing to restore order crossed the Nu Jiang river, also known as Thanlwin in Burmese and Salween in English. This is a mighty watercourse, running for 1,500 miles from its source in Tibet to the estuary in Myanmar's Gulf of Mottama. Its upper reaches constituted a barrier between rodents carrying bubonic plague and non-infected species on the other side. The returning Chinese troops were unaware that infected rodents crossed the river with them, and thus brought the plague into China. Forty years later the epidemic reached European communities in Shanghai and Hong Kong, horrifying the expats there and drawing the attention of European researchers like those in Paris at the Institut Pasteur, founded by Louis Pasteur in 1887. By training a biologist and microbiologist, he made a number of discoveries of great importance in the unending fight against disease, reducing mortality from puerperal fever that killed so many women after childbirth and creating the first vaccines for rabies and anthrax. Best known today for his work in pasteurising milk and wine, he was buried in a vault beneath the institute, but post mortem examination of his notebooks revealed that this paragon of scientific virtue also cheated at times to stay ahead of his rivals.

One of those was the German physician and microbiologist Robert Koch (1843–1910). He identified the causes of tuberculosis, cholera and anthrax. For his work on tuberculosis he received a Nobel Prize. In his work on anthrax he formulated a set of four postulates, which may sound common sense today, but were important for tightening up the conditions of serious research into disease at a time when contamination skewed many researchers' results:

1. The suspected pathogen must be present in every case of the disease.
2. The organism must be taken from a diseased host and grown in a pure culture medium.

3. Samples of the organism taken from the pure culture must cause the same disease when inoculated into a healthy, susceptible experimental animal.
4. The organism must then be isolated from the inoculated animal and be identified as the same organism originally isolated from the first diseased host.

The plague bacillus causing bubonic plague remained a mystery until identified in 1894 by a Swiss researcher who had worked under Pasteur. Alexandre Yersin (1863–1943) arrived in Hong Kong three days after Japanese pathologist Shibasaburo Kitasato, famous for the discovery of the role of *clostridium tetani* in lockjaw. Kitasato having already acquired by bribery exclusive access to all the available corpses of plague victims in the colony, Yersin had to bribe two British sailors working between ships as orderlies in the hospital morgue to let him take samples of the contents of the victims' buboes, which Kitasato had ignored. Yersin's method was to puncture with a sterile pipette a swollen lymph node of a patient who had just died. Under his microscope, he was able to see in the aspirate some small gram-negative bacilli with rounded ends. He injected this into mice and guinea pigs, which quickly died. Two days later he informed the British authorities in Hong Kong of his findings. Later, it would be known that there are eleven species in the *yersinia* genus, which originated 3,335 years ago. So far, only three of these have been able to infect humans: *Y. pestis, Y. enterocolitica* and *Y. pseudotuberculosis.*

However, both *The Lancet* and the *British Medical Journal* had already credited Kitasato with the discovery of the cause of bubonic plague on the basic of his cultures, which were contaminated by pneumococci. So Yersin informed the Académie de Sciences in Paris. When the two British journals printed Yersin's letter, it became apparent that Kitasato had failed to find the real cause of the plague, and Yersin received the due credit. He named the bacillus *Pasteurella pestis*, after his mentor, Louis Pasteur. Half a century later in 1944, the name was changed to *Yersinia pestis*.[1] It is interesting that Yersin missed the all-important vectors of the plague, understanding nothing of the importance of rats and fleas. This was discovered independently by Dr Masanori Ogata in Formosa and a medically trained missionary named Paul Louis Simond in Bombay.

Yersin's plague reached Bombay in 1898 and claimed 10 million lives in the sub-continent during the next decade. Carried by international trade, this plague spread to South Africa, and both South and North America. In each case, it established reservoirs of infection in rodent species. Not all were burrowers; in California they were ground squirrels, who spread the focus north to Canada and south into Mexico. Now, in the USA plague is carried by no fewer than thirty-four species of rodents and thirty-five species of fleas can act as vectors.[2] Experiments have shown that, even after rodents have left a complex of burrows, *Y.Pestis* can survive in the soil for nearly a year, infecting yet another generation of tunneling rodents who move in to exploit the same territory.

On 3 August 1900 bubonic plague visited Glasgow. At first being mis-identified as typhoid, it affected thirty-six people, of whom sixteen died. One of the doctors treating the victims pushed his investigations further, and concluded that they were suffering from bubonic plague. The official report of the Local Government Board for Scotland hypothesised that foreign sailors using the city's brothels were passing the disease to prostitutes. But Glasgow's own public health officers sent numerous rat-catchers into the crowded tenements of the Gorbals and found in dissected rats symptoms of the disease.

Various species of rats, by the way, have been responsible for infecting humans with several killer diseases, as have guinea pigs, rabbits and even tiny harvest mice. The vector is often tinier mites, transferring typhus to field workers, and from them into the general population. Tick bites also transfer typhus and the ticks can transfer the disease between generations, so that no animal reservoir is necessary. In Europe, however, it is usually lice that infect the victims. Similar to typhus are the Japanese Tsutsugamushi fever and the Rocky Mountain spotted fever in the USA. There is even a version of European typhus named Brill's disease because it was identified in 1898 among immigrants in New York by a physician of that name.

A mystery remained as to who had introduced the plague to Glasgow until she was identified as a fish-wife, who met many people every day at the fish market. Whether or not she also worked on the side as a prostitute, is unknown, but either way it seems she may have initially contracted the infection from a fisherman or sailor from elsewhere.[3] During this short-duration plague, there were calls for disinfecting all the trams and ferries and all the coins in circulation, in case they carried the infection. The Catholic Church agreed to prohibit temporarily the customary wakes after a death, to avoid too many people getting together and infecting each other.[4]

Yersin and Kitasato were not the only ones searching for the cause of fatal diseases in 1894. Waldemar Haffkine (1860–1930), known as the vaccine pioneer the world forgot, was a 33-year-old émigré Russian who was in Calcutta. From the moment he arrived there, he was made unwelcome both by the British medical establishment and the native population. Apart from being Jewish, he had trained in Odessa and worked in Paris not as a doctor but a zoologist. There, he had developed what he hoped would be a reliable vaccine for cholera. In his first year in India, he vaccinated 23,000 people in the north of the country, many of whom did not return for the second injection, one week after the first. Also, although millions in the sub-continent had cholera, none of his patients seemed to come into contact with it.

In March of 1894 he was invited to Calcutta by the British medical officer of the city in order to track down the source of cholera in some of the *bustees* or primitive villages near the city where the inhabitants all shared the same unclean and inadequate water source. Haffkine travelled to a *bustee* named Kattal Bagan and vaccinated 116 of the 200 inhabitants. Among the unvaccinated half of the village there were nine fatalities, but none among the people he had vaccinated. The Calcutta medical officer of health was impressed enough to finance a bigger trial but few Indians trusted the idea of vaccination, thinking that the British administration of the Raj was trying to poison them. To overcome their resistance, Haffine vaccinated himself, but few were convinced.

Perhaps because of his frustration with the cholera vaccine, Haffkine turned to what he hoped would be a single-injection vaccine for the plague, which was endemic in the sub-continent. An experiment with rabbits was successful, so he injected himself with three times the dose he thought necessary and succumbed to a high fever, but recovered in a few days. In January 1897 he used an outbreak of plague in a Bombay prison as a field trial, vaccinating 147 prisoners and leaving 172 as a control group. Among the unvaccinated there were twelve cases of plague, six of them fatal. Among the vaccinated, there were two cases of infection, but no deaths.

Moving into far superior accommodation provided by the grateful government, Haffkine was delighted that the Aga Khan, leader of the

Ismaili Muslims, volunteered himself and all the members of his sect for vaccination. Hundreds of thousands of lives being saved by Haffkine's plague vaccine, he was knighted and promoted to the post of director of the Plague Research laboratory in Mumbai with fifty-three people working under him. Just when it seemed that he would be known as the saviour of India came a disaster with nineteen people dying in the Punjab among 107 treated with Haffkine's tetanus vaccine. The deaths were traced to one contaminated bottle of vaccine from his laboratory in Mumbai. Haffkine was sacked.

In disgrace, Haffkine travelled to London, and was still there, trying to clear his name, two years later when plague killed more than a million people in India. In 1906 the British government of India finally published the result of a commission of inquiry, finding Haffkine guilty of malpractice for the Punjab tetanus deaths. A professor at King's College in London presented a detailed exoneration of Haffkine and blamed the poor hygiene of an assistant performing the vaccination, when a pair of forceps fell to the floor and were used without sterilisation. The professor was joined by Dr Ronald Ross, the Nobel laureate knighted for his work on the transmission of malaria, and pioneer bacteriologist Lord Lister also praised Haffkine as the saviour of mankind. As a result, he was reinstated as head of the Calcutta biological laboratory, but allowed only to do theoretical research. Retiring early, he died in Lausanne in 1930 at the age of 70. In 1964, the Indian government honoured the man who had saved so many lives with his portrait on a postage stamp.

Twelve plague outbreaks in Australia between 1900 and 1925 managed to kill off only 1,000 people, most of them in Sydney. The San Francisco plague of 1900–04 was followed by another outbreak in 1907–08. In 1911 and 1921 new outbreaks of plague from the original reservoir among Central Asian rodents occurred in Manchuria. The nomads who formerly lived there had a taboo about touching or catching marmots, and would even move their encampments away if obviously sick marmots were found nearby. In 1911 as the Manchu dynasty collapsed, the consequent end of the former embargo on ethnic Chinese moving into the plague area and trapping tarabagan marmots for their fur, some of them infected, produced an epidemic.

Currently there are eleven species that comprise the *Yersinia* genus, of which only three can infect humans. Its bubonic form is the most common and is generally transmitted subcutaneously to a human host through a vector like an infected flea. The pathogen reproduces and within days after infection an individual will experience the formation of buboes (swollen lymph nodes) across the surface of the skin, while the disease simultaneously spreads via the bloodstream to other organs, such as the liver and spleen where it causes further damage to tissues.

A victim contracts *Y. enterocolitica* by consuming infected food or water, leading speedily to gastroenteritis.[5] The two other forms of *Y. pestis* infection, septicaemic and pneumonic, remain less common. The pneumonic does not require an arthropod-vector like a rat flea for transmission because the infection is carried into the lungs by cough droplets from someone already infected. It then clogs the lungs with bodily fluids, making it impossible to breathe and causing death in as little as twenty-four hours. The brief period within which it kills has led some scholars to claim *Y. pestis* as the deadliest known pathogen. Whole-genome research suggests that all lineages of *Y. pestis* are descended from an ancient *Y. pseudotuberculosis* line[6] and there are fears that it may develop a resistance to antibiotics.

This pathogen since resurfaced in Uganda causing pneumonic plague in 2004. In 2005–06, 204 cases of this plague were reported in the Democratic Republic of Congo and in 2014 sixty victims died in northern Madagascar. There, two young brothers, working in a copper mine in Beramanja, set out on 6 January to walk thirty-five miles to their family home in Ankatakata. Somewhere on the journey, they picked up the infection. The 13-year-old developed fever, headache, and chills with severe chest pain and the coughing up of blood. He died at the family home on 14 January. On 21 January his mother, who had nursed him until he died, also died. His father, a daughter and a granddaughter all died on the following day.

The people living in single-room houses, the circumstances in the Madagascar outbreak are similar to those of medieval and earlier plagues in Europe. Friends and neighbours who cared for the victims carried the plague to four other villages by 9 February. After plague arrived, probably from India, at the port of Toamasina in 1898, the Madagascan personnel of Institut Pasteur in Antananarivo was assigned to control this disease. They were instrumental in stopping the 2014 outbreak with relatively few fatalities. However, because of the remoteness of the affected villages, fifteen victims died before they could have treatment, one boy after carrying his infected sister several miles to a traditional healer. She died, as did two others taken to traditional healers. Health care professionals arrived on 28 January, but some contacts refused chemoprophylaxis and died anyway. Five victims who received streptomycin survived. Difficulty of access and severe weather prevented any investigation until 1 April, when sixty-four rodents were trapped, none of them showing infection, although in the central highland rain forests of Madagascar and in the Congo and Peru there are known foci of infection. WHO reported 320 cases worldwide in 2017, causing seventy-seven deaths.

At the same time, our old enemy influenza was biding its time. In 1957–58 an Asian 'flu virus, thought to have originated in birds or pigs, caused between 1.5 and 2 million deaths worldwide. In 1957 a global network of laboratories linked to the World Influenza Research Centre in London, founded as a clearing house for research and tracking the virus. The quarterly report of the British Public Health Laboratory Service mentioned in March 1957 that seasonal 'flu had caused a *low* level of respiratory illness that winter. Yet a *Times* newspaper article of 17 April mentioned that a new strain of the virus had affected thousands of Hong Kong residents, who had no immunity to it. The flood gates were open. By mid-May there were 100,000 victims in Taiwan. Over 1 million were laid low in India by June as the virus went on a world tour. Early in 1958 it was estimated 9 million people in Great Britain – half of them under the age of 14 – had, or had had, the symptoms of unsteadiness, exhaustion, sore throat, coughs, pain in the limbs and head and high fever. Symptoms peaked in two waves, the second a week or two after the first. Yet, only 14,000 deaths were recorded in Britain as being directly attributable to this H1N1 virus. Some general practitioners prescribed penicillin or other antibiotics to calm their patients; while these had no effect on the viral pneumonia, they did act on any secondary bacterial pneumonia. In Britain, an appeal was broadcast, asking the public not to visit the doctor if they felt 'flu coming on but to stay at home and take aspirin. After some ten years of evolution, this variant virus seemingly disappeared, being replaced through antigenic shift by a new influenza A subtype, labelled H3N2. This in turn gave us the 1968 Hong Kong 'flu pandemic, which caused another million deaths.

Closer to today, in January 2009, another 'flu virus emerged in North America and lasted to August 2010 after infecting maybe a fifth of the human race. It contained a combination of influenza genes not previously known in humans and was designated as an influenza A (H1N1)pdm09.

Although the elderly had antibodies from earlier encounters with the old H1N1, the young were particularly affected by the new virus. In twelve months, the US Centre for Disease Control (CDC) estimated there had been 60.8 million cases with a quarter-million hospitalisations and 12,469 deaths. H1N1pdm09 continues as a seasonal flu virus, causing illness, hospitalisation, and deaths worldwide every year. With the official designation hard to memorise, not surprisingly it became known colloquially as swine 'flu, referring to its origin as a reassortment of bird, swine and human 'flu viruses, complicated by a Eurasian pig virus.

Was that the full story? Not really. It was eventually concluded that between 284,500 and 579,000 people could have been killed by the disease, but the majority of these fatalities were guesswork because they occurred in Africa and southeast Asia, where there were no facilities to compile statistics. A subsequent report compiled by researchers in 2016 at the Mount Sinai School of Medicine in New York was that the 2009 H1N1 virus probably originated from factory-farmed pigs in central Mexico, its first human victim a 5-year-old boy at La Gloria, a rural town in Mexico's Veracruz state. So, all in all 'swine fever' was a reasonable name for the outbreak. Various health agencies advised that properly cooked pork presented no risk to the consumer, but the Indonesian government halted the importation of pigs and required the extermination of 9 million pigs in that predominantly Muslim country. In Cairo the government went a step further, ordering the slaughter of all the pigs in Egypt. That's a lot of bacon going up in smoke.

Chapter 12

Sundry Fevers and the Spanish 'flu

Although now mainly confined to tropical Third World countries, malaria has been known for many centuries since being mentioned in Chinese archives as particularly affecting non-Chinese invaders from the north who had no previous exposure to it, and therefore no immunity. Hippocrates, the father of Greek medicine, lived probably 460-377 BCE. He recorded an epidemic of mumps on the island of Thasos[1] and three-day and four-day fevers that are thought likely to have been tertian and quartan malarial fever.[2]

Malaria was rampant in Europe during the twelfth century when Eleanor of Aquitaine and her first husband Louis VII of France visited Rome on their way home from the Second Crusade. Although this very religious French king was unable to resist a side-trip to Rome in all its medieval squalor so that he could pray at the graves of several apostles, Eleanor managed to hurry him swiftly away to avoid the fever long attributed to *la mal'aria* or bad air from swamps of the *campagna*, to which the locals seemed to have developed a measure of immunity.[3]

King Richard the Lionheart, her most famous son fathered by her second husband King Henry II of England, had suffered malaria – then endemic in Europe – before setting off on the Third Crusade. In the Holy Land he caught a possibly viral and very infectious fever called *arnaldia* – as did the French king, Philippe Auguste. For a time, both these leaders of the crusade were *hors de combat*.[4] After crusaders brought the disease back to Europe on their return, it was known in France as *la suette* and in England as 'the sweating syknes'. Apart from debilitating sweats, the symptoms included skin rashes, the nails and hair falling out, lips peeling painfully and whole strips of skin falling away from the body. After reappearing in 1502, 1508, 1517, 1528 and 1551, it last appeared in northern France in 1906. One victim of the 1502 outbreak was Arthur, Prince of Wales, whose death enabled his younger brother to succeed their father Henry VII on the throne. Crowned as Henry VIII, the surviving brother was a very different monarch than Arthur would have been.

Five centuries later Emperor Napoléon III sent the French Foreign Legion across the Atlantic as France's contribution to the ill-fated *affaire mexicana*, which aimed to impose the Austrian emperor's brother Prince Maximilian as ruler of Mexico. The legionnaires, despite their recent experience of war in the Crimea and Italy, were not sent to besiege the capital city, but tasked with securing the *camino real* between the port of Vera Cruz and Mexico city because they were not French and could be written off with no political repercussions in France. Patrolling the *camino real* was not a job one would wish on a friend because the coastal area through which it passed had just about all the unpleasant diseases of the tropics including a variant of yellow fever called *vómito negro* in which the victims vomited up their own blood for six or eight hours before dying with agonising cramps. Not everybody caught this, but every man suffered malaria. So called 'Jesuits' powder' – the powdered bark of the cinchona tree – was known to cure this and had been used in Europe for two centuries, saving the life of England's Charles II among other important people. Nobody was about to waste this expensive medication on the legionnaires, so they suffered recurrent fevers and died by the dozen.[5]

Not until twenty years later, when French army doctor Alphonse Laveran published his *Traité des fièvres palustres* in 1884 was it realised that the cause of malaria was the *plasmodium* parasite. In the following year, British army officer Dr Ronald Ross, who was suffering malaria himself in India despite daily prophylactic doses of quinine, observed under the microscope some early-stage plasmodium parasites in the stomach of a female anopheles mosquito, and the circle was complete. Later knighted for his work, Ross correctly deduced how these mosquitoes transferred the *plasmodium* pathogen to their human victims.

Another French researcher named Paul-Louis Symond found by using a more powerful microscope in 1898 that the proliferating bacteria block the throat of the infected mosquito, which attempts to avoid starvation by regurgitating the bacteria when injecting blood-thinning agents to facilitate sucking blood from its human victim through its very narrow stylets. These mosquitoes can also transmit West Nile virus, dengue fever, yellow fever and other diseases in the same way. From 1926 and especially during the enormous movements of troops into the tropics during the Second World War, quinine was replaced as a prophylactic by atabrine under various proprietorial names. This was itself later replaced as a treatment for malaria by chloroquine, the drug which US President Trump decided on no scientific basis would cure Coved-19 during the 2019–21 pandemic.

The last pandemic of the nineteenth century is still a mystery. It had a name: Russian flu, because it was first reported in May 1889 in the Central Asian city-state of Bokhara, then within the tsarist Russian empire, where it killed two-thirds of all infected people. Travelling along the Trans-Caspian railway, the mystery pathogen sped 3,300 kilometres to Siberian Omsk in three months before using the trade route along the Volga river to reach St Petersburg and Kiev in the Ukraine that November. Then the capital of Russia, St Petersburg had been built on the Baltic by Peter the Great expressly to connect with the European states by water. From Scandinavia, the Russian 'flu reached every European capital by December, and leaped the Atlantic, covering the USA and as far south as Argentina in February 1989. Within the twelvemonth it had infected the entire inhabited planet. Unbelievably, contemporary professors of medicine announced that it was not contagious, but spread by miasmas and treatable with quinine, strychnine or whiskey and brandy.

Russian 'flu killed about 1 million people worldwide, the most vulnerable being the very young, the old, and those with pre-existing health problems. The specific cause of death was usually pneumonia or a heart attack brought on by the physical stress of fighting for breath. But as to what the specific pathogen was, researchers differ. Some say it was a virus designated A/H2N2; others label it virus A/HeN8; still others consider it was a coronavirus designated OC43, possibly a mutated form of a bovine coronavirus. The main waves of the infection were May 1889–December 1890, March–June 1891, November 1891–June 1892 and winter 1893–early 1895, but within these times there were periods when infection lessened, for reasons unknown.

Researchers have tried for many years to identify the subtypes of Influenza A responsible for the 1889–91, 1898–1900 and 1918 epidemics. Initially, this work was primarily based on 'seroarcheology' – the detection of antibodies to influenza infection in the sera of elderly people – and it was thought that the 1889–91 pandemic was caused by Influenza A subtype H2, which killed 100,000 in the US and was thought at the time to have been brought to America by the thousands of poor immigrants from Eastern Europe crossing the Atlantic in steerage on steamships. It is now thought that it originated in South China, although known at the time as Russian 'flu, which killed 100,000 in Britain. Later, the epidemics of 1898–1900 were attributed to subtype H3, and the 1918 pandemic by subtype H1. With the confirmation of H1N1 as the cause of the 1918 'flu pandemic following identification of H1N1 antibodies in exhumed corpses, re-analysis of seroarcheological data has indicated that Influenza A subtype H3 (possibly the H3N8 subtype), is a more likely cause for the 1889–90 pandemic.

In early 1918, as the war in the trenches ground bloodily on, a particularly fatal form of influenza added its crop of lives to that of the war 'in Flanders fields', the intensively manured soil of which was rich in human and animal excrement and human and equine body parts rendered too small by high explosives, or too deeply buried, to be removed. In Britain, where health statistics were reasonably accurate, it was estimated that this 'flu killed 250,000 civilians and 400,000 civilians in France. Elsewhere, the statistics are vague; the war was killing millions; millions more were starving as normal food production failed; in large areas of Africa and Asia there was no government machinery to record civilian deaths, although British India counted 20 million deaths.

Notwithstanding still being called 'Spanish flu' today, this pandemic did not originate on the Iberian peninsula. So why the name? Isolated physically from the rest of Europe by the Pyrenees, with few terrestrial links to its nearest neighbour France, Spain remained neutral in the First World War, as it would in 1939–45. It therefore had no comprehensive press censorship, unlike the belligerent states, whose governments strictly limited what news could and could not be reported in the media of the day. In the absence of other reporting of the pandemic, the news coming out of Spain as the 'flu spread unfortunately earned for the Iberian nation the ownership of this scourge. It was also referred to as 'the Spanish Lady' and depicted in cartoons as a gaunt flamenco dancer with a death's head playing the part of a prostitute who infected fatally all she touched. Call it what you will, the thing to remember about the H1N1A virus that caused all the deaths is that, after laying low for nine decades, in 2009 it returned, modified by elements of avian, human and pig pathogens, the last earning it the common name 'swine 'flu.' For nineteen months, the pandemic raged quietly across the planet, causing 284,000 deaths according to WHO.

Yet today this is virtually forgotten, unlike the original outbreak of the Spanish 'flu, which lasted from February 1918 to April 1920. It apparently began at Camp Kearney in California, and next appeared at Camp Funston in Kansas when a US army cook named Albert Gitchell reported sick on 4 March 1918. At first the medical officer attributed his breathing difficulties to a severe dust storm the previous day. By the end of that sick call, dozens of others were in the sick bay with the same symptoms. Credit is due to Dr Loring Miner, who practised medicine in Haskell County, Kansas, for warning the US Public Health Service that this was no ordinary influenza. Within a week 522 men had reported sick at Camp Funston with the same symptoms as the cook. Men were also falling ill at Fort Riley in Kansas. Since the virus reached New York within a few weeks, it seems that no quarantine was enforced in Kansas by the US army medical services.

Camp Funston was a major training facility for troops destined to be sent to the American Expeditionary Forces in France. Since the United States had only entered the war in April 1917, by when the European allies had been fighting Germany and Austro-Hungary for two and a half years, the recruitment and training of American conscripts was under considerable pressure. Intakes of new recruits arrived at the camp every week and trained troops passed out at the end of their time there, like a production line in a factory. It was just the place to give the pathogen H1N1A a perfect start.

In September, when Surgeon-General Victor Vaughan was ordered to Camp Devens near Boston, Massachusetts, he arrived to see hundreds of young men crowding into wards where every bed was already occupied. Their faces, he noted, wore a bluish cast and they were coughing up bloody sputum. That day sixty-three men died. Vaughan also noted that, while most influenza outbreaks carried off the old and the very young, the new strain aimed particularly at those in the prime of life.

The infection went epidemic in the American Midwest and the East Coast ports from which the men were shipped to Europe. President Wilson was advised of the situation and had to decide between quarantining hundreds of thousands of men on American soil until the epidemic died down – if it did – and acceding to the demands of US Expeditionary Forces commander-in-chief General John Joseph Pershing, nicknamed Black Jack. Pershing insisted that he needed hundreds of thousands more men to replace the daily toll of casualties, and was aware that many of the reinforcements would be unfit for combat duty because they had received little real training. President Wilson chose to prioritise the war.

There were no purpose-built troopships to transport the reinforcements across the Atlantic, so civilian ships, including confiscated German vessels, were hastily converted and the men crammed into them, sweating in three-tier bunks below decks with poor ventilation. Again, this was exactly what the virus needed; the ships were effectively incubation chambers, as were the cruise ships immobilised in various ports with quarantined passengers confined to their cabins for weeks during the 2020 coronavirus pandemic. On the troopship USS *Leviathan* in September 1918, ninety-six men died during the crossing. On disembarkation at the French port of Brest, the infected survivors passed the virus to dock workers who spread it more widely throughout France, and from there to Spain and Italy. Before the end of April 1917, men were falling ill all along the Western Front. British casualties with a 'Blighty wound' meriting repatriation and officers on leave carried it to England. In France, immense military hospitals had to be improvised, far larger than those made for the steady stream of casualties, which never killed as many as the 'flu. One might think that the zone of active hostilities would constitute a fire-break, but cases started appearing in the German lines too, having possibly travelled via a roundabout route through neutral Switzerland. Eventually nearly a million German personnel were unfit to fight, as were half the British Tommies and two-thirds of the French *poilus* in Flanders.

Whatever its route, H1N1A reached Poland in May and continued to Odessa in Russia. After all the mutinies in the tsarist forces on the eastern fronts leading to complete collapse, the Bolshevik government had signed the treaty of Brest-Litovsk on 3 March and several million Russian POWS were being shipped East by the Central Powers to end the need for their captors to feed and guard them. With these men, from the Polish frontier to far Siberia, travelled the virus. In May it reached North Africa, India, southeast Asia, China and Japan. By July it had reached Australia, which had applied very strict quarantine restrictions on ships coming from overseas, so perhaps it was carried there with shipments of wounded soldiers returning from Europe. Strangely enough, this first wave of infections did not appear to be very dangerous. Ignoring war casualties in Flanders, not many more people died in the first six months of 1918 than in the same period of the previous year, and most of the fatalities were of the elderly or people with pre-existing health problems. But by the end of the outbreak the virus had infected an estimated 500 million people or one-third of the world's population, causing death in – statistics vary – between 50 and 100 million victims. Among the unpleasant symptoms of the infection was bleeding from the mucous membrane of the nose, mouth, throat, respiratory tract and intestines.

In the Western Hemisphere, a second wave of the pandemic started in late August, radiating outwards from Boston, Massachusetts to cover the Eastern seaboard of the US and then virtually all North America in the following couple of months. In those days when children made their own amusements, girls particularly enjoyed skipping to the rhythm of songs. A new skipping song 'went viral' as one might say today:

> I had a little bird.
> Its name was Enza.
> I opened the window
> And in flew Enza.

Having reached the borders of the USA, it continued north into Canada and southward into Central and South America and the Caribbean. At the same time, in Africa it radiated outward from Freetown in Liberia, to reach Ethiopia on the other side of the continent in November. In Eurasia, this wave used First World War Russian troop movements along the Trans-Siberian railway to reach the Pacific coast, meeting up in northern Russia with the infection brought by troops of the Allied interventionist forces landed at Archangelsk in Russia's far north.[6] It was hard not to see the virus as a malignant creature, whose tentacles reached south through Central Asia to hit India and Iran in September and China and Japan in November, by which point it covered all the inhabited continents. Yet, by the end of the year, it seemed to be dying out.

What were the symptoms in 1918? At first, the usual ones of influenza: sore throat, headaches and fever, but in the second wave, many weakened sufferers contracted a bacterial infection on top of the flu and died in hours or a couple of days, drowned by the build-up of yellowish purulent secretions in their lungs, uncovered in autopsies. Some victims who had recovered from the first wave seemed to have acquired a degree of immunity, suggesting that this was the same virus, and the quasi-immunity of older people may have been due to having acquired a degree of immunity by exposure to the pandemic of Russian 'flu in 1889–90.

After the October 1917 Revolution in Russia, the vast extent of the former tsarist empire was in chaos from the Baltic Sea to the Pacific Ocean and from the Black Sea to the frozen expanse of the White Sea. The entire infrastructure of what came to be called euphemistically 'the Socialist sixth of the world' collapsed with millions killed fighting the Germans and Austrians in the First World War followed by uncounted millions more in a civil war between the Russian White, or pro-tsarist, forces reinforced by interventionist contingents sent by foreign governments against Trotsky's Red Army. Typhus was already endemic in Russia before the Revolution and later expanded into an epidemic concurrent with the Spanish 'flu, infecting an estimated 30 million cases in the malnourished or starving population, of whom 3 million men, women and children died from this cause.

Whereas the first planet-wide wave of H1N1A had targeted the sick and elderly, the second one killed the young and healthy. It has been suggested that this may have been because soldiers with mild symptoms 'just carried on' with their duties, while those with severe symptoms were transported *en masse* to hospitals, where they effectively passed on their infections or acquired worse ones. It is also theorised that many soldiers' lungs, already damaged by exposure to gas warfare, were unable to cope with the infection. In the last quarter of 1918 nearly 300,000 died in the USA. Even this was nothing compared with the estimates of related deaths in India, which ranged from 12.5 to 20 million. Something happened to the virus at the end of the year because a third wave of infections in 1919 was less severe, but still widespread enough to be a global emergency, killing hundreds of thousands in Spain, Mexico, Serbia and Britain and tens of thousands in the USA during the first half of 1919. In late 1919 and the spring of 1920, a fourth wave occurred very unevenly, hitting Switzerland, Scandinavia, Peru and Japan with renewed virulence.

At the time, the virus H1N1A was too small to be seen by the best optical microscopes then available. The immensely more powerful – and vastly more expensive – electron microscopes were not available until 1938. Because researchers at the time of the 1918 pandemic could see through their optical microscopes a bacterium named *haemophilus influenzae* in samples taken from many victims it was thought that this was the cause of the pandemic. There were, of course, no antibiotics to fight the virus, once installed in a patient's body, but there was a vaccine for *h. influenzae* which did cure some victims, if it was administered in time, but that was only acting on the secondary infection. Some medical professionals became convinced that the killer disease was typhus, which was indeed rampant in Russia, torn by the civil war. Some others administered Epsom salts, quinine, aspirin, arsenic, castor oil or iodine taken internally, with results unknown.

Some geographically isolated territories like Australia and Iceland introduced strict quarantines, but even more isolated New Zealand failed to impose quarantine on ships leaving port and spreading the infection to a number of the Pacific islands, although German-occupied Samoa was saved by its quarantine. As in 2020, social distancing was imposed in some countries, where schools and theatres were closed, and face masks were used in certain countries too, although, as in 2020, many people in the USA refused to wear them, copying US President Donald Trump, even when attending rallies with thousands of supporters. He paid the price of ignorance and arrogance, reporting sick with Covid-19 in early October 2020.

Where did H1N1A come from? Studies in various countries have confirmed that it originated in North America, alternatively that it manifested itself spontaneously in war-torn Europe or that it came from China with the tens of thousands of coolies transported to the Western Front to serve in the labour corps. You can take your pick. It seems that some research establishments do just that, apparently for political reasons. For example, some researchers believed that the German drug company Bayer had poisoned all its aspirin tablets sold internationally with H1N1A. Almost inevitably, the miasma theory resurfaced, this time blaming the gases of decomposition of millions of corpses in the mass graves under Flanders fields and elsewhere.

Chapter 13

Covid-19 Emerges

Although most people might say that had never heard the term 'coronavirus' before the 2020 pandemic, 20 per cent of the millions who have had a common cold owed their sniffles and congestion to one. Of the others, 60 per cent were suffering from a rhinovirus or other kind of known virus and the last 20 per cent were suffering from an unidentified virus. All of this explains why there is not much point in expecting the doctor to cure a cold. He or she may prescribe an antibiotic, but this will have no effect on the cause of the cold, although it may stave off opportunistic bacteria taking advantage of the weakened state of the cold victim.

Although recognised as a medical condition for a century, the common cold is still without a cure, despite causing the loss of millions of work days each year and seriously exacerbating conditions like chronic obstructive pulmonary disease and cystic fibrosis when patients with these problems also get a cold. In the United States it is estimated that 100 million doctor visits annually are due to the common cold. Sufferers spend annually $3 billion on over-the-counter and $400 millions on prescription drugs that may relieve some symptoms without curing the cold. Part of the problem in making a vaccine is that colds may be caused by any of 200 different viruses, mostly rhinoviruses, but also some coronaviruses. Of these, HCoV-OC43, HKU1 and HCoV-229E cause mild upper-respiratory illness; HCoV-NL63 can cause croup and bronchiolitis in children. Three others – SARS-CoV, MERS-CoV and SARS-CoV2 – are potential killers of infected humans.

Virologists have known about coronaviruses since the 1960s. Technically, they are enveloped positive stranded members of the *nidovirales* group whose reservoirs of infection are in animals as varied as bats and pigs. When first examined through an electron microscope, they appeared to be disc-shaped with spikes sticking out all round. Hence the name incorporating the Latin *corona*, which can mean a crown or halo. If examined in three dimensions, they can be seen as spherical with protein spikes sticking out in all directions. It is these spikes that pierce body cells' defences and 'unlock' the cells for the virus to invade.

Identified in November 2002, SARS-CoV earned its initials by causing severe acute respiratory syndrome. Carried by international travellers, it rapidly spread from China to twenty-six other countries. In one documented case a Chinese-American businessman flew from China to Vietnam on 26 February 2003, not aware he had SARS. Two days later he was hospitalised at the Hanoi French Hospital with severe respiratory problems, dying there on 6 March after infecting hospital staff. SARS arrived in Canada on 5 March with an elderly Chinese-Canadian woman and her husband who, during a visit to Hong Kong, had been staying in a hotel on Kowloon side 18-21 February. On 6 March SARS arrived in Singapore with three passengers from Hong Kong; on 10 March it was in Taipei, capital of Taiwan; on 15 March it landed in Germany with a doctor who had been treating patients in Singapore; on 18 March it arrived in Manchester with a man from Hong Kong. On 25 March the pathogen was identified as a new coronavirus – only the second known, the first being variants of the coronaviruses that cause the common cold.[1]

Fortunately, the SARS outbreak in Toronto is well documented. The Chinese woman felt ill after her return from Hong Kong on 23 February and was cared for at home by family members, including her adult son. He became Case A, falling ill on 27 February and reporting to hospital as an emergency with severe respiratory symptoms on 7 March. Placed in an observation facility after eighteen hours, he had already infected two other patients in the emergency ward. After eighteen hours, Case A was placed in airborne isolation because it appeared possible that he had tuberculosis. On 12 March WHO issued a worldwide alert about a severe respiratory syndrome spreading among hospital care workers in Hanoi, Vietnam, and Hong Kong. After this alert was forwarded to Toronto, on 13 March, contact and droplet isolation precautions were imposed in the ICU, although Case A's family members were allowed to visit. After having chest x-rays, four of them were instructed to wear masks at all times and limit their visits to the ICU, washing their hands on each occasion.

Case A died that day, by which time several other family members had breathing difficulties.

Case B became febrile on 10 March, three days after exposure to Case A in the emergency department. Somebody in Toronto reasoned that the family's health problems might be linked to the cases of atypical pneumonia being reported in Hong Kong. Four members of the family were admitted to three different hospitals on 13 March, and one more was admitted to hospital on the following day, all subject to airborne, droplet, and contact precautions. Case B was brought to the index hospital on 16 March by two emergency paramedics, who did not use special precautions. After nine hours isolated in the emergency department, Case B was transferred to the ICU. His wife became ill on 16 March and visited him in the ICU on 21 March before he died later that day. Three other members of case B's extended family also developed SARS, as did the paramedics who brought Case B to the hospital, a firefighter, five emergency department staff, one other member of staff, two patients in the emergency ward and a housekeeper who worked there. Seven visitors to the emergency ward while Case B was there suffered symptoms beginning 19-26 March. All these in turn transmitted the infection to sixteen other contacts. In the ICU, Case B was intubated for mechanical ventilation by a doctor wearing his usual surgical mask, gown and gloves, which gave no protection. He also acquired SARS and transmitted it to a member of his family. Three ICU nurses attending the intubation using droplet and contact precautions suffered symptoms between 18-20 March, one transmitting the infection to a household member.

Case C was admitted to the index hospital on 13 March after a heart attack. It was not known that he had been in contact with case A on 7 March, so no one realised he also had SARS. No precautions being taken, he spent three days in the coronary care unit and was then transferred for renal dialysis to another hospital, where he died on 29 March after infecting seventeen members of staff at the index hospital, a paramedic and several patients. These in turn infected hospital staff and family members. Case C's wife became ill on 26 March, by which date the scale of the emergency was realised. Additional isolation facilities were requisitioned, but all the hospitals in Toronto could only scape together enough qualified staff to handle fourteen more SARS patients. The government of Ontario attacked the crisis, ordering all hospitals in the province to prepare units for SARS patients. In addition to nineteen confirmed cases in Canada – one 2,000 miles away in Vancouver – and to suspend 'non-essential' admissions. Personal protection equipment was to be supplied to all exposed staff, but it took time before some one realised how the infection travelled through the hospitals' air conditioning systems and the importance of negative air pressure in the treatment rooms to counteract this.

On 14 May WHO removed Toronto from the list of danger areas, signifying that the outbreak was ended. The state of emergency ended on 17 May with 140 probable and 178 suspect infections. Twenty-four patients had died, all in Ontario. But by 9 June seventy-nine previously unidentified cases of SARS had been identified. Overall, the fatality rate was 9.6 percent, with advanced age the most important risk factor; patients older than 60 having a fatality rate of 45 per cent. Other high risk categories are patients with diabetes and hepatitis B. Even 9.6 per cent fatality was a high rate. Researchers at the National Institute of Allergy and Infectious Diseases (NIAID) in Bethesda, Maryland, and Hamilton, Montana, immediately leaped into action, studying this coronavirus and developing a DVA vaccine candidate for it. For a while, it seemed that Irish humourist Spike Milligan (1918–2002) had been ahead of the field in stating that unpleasant 'diseases that attack people's kneeses ... come from the East wrapped in bladders of yeast, so the Chinese must take all the blame'.[2]

But then in September 2012 a similar disease appeared in the Middle East and was dubbed MERS-CoV, standing for Middle East Respiratory Syndrome. This is an illness caused by the coronavirus MERS-Cov, which originated in the Arabian peninsula, where it was first reported in Saudi Arabia, but subsequent research indicated its occurrence in Jordan five months earlier. Although the largest reported outbreak was in Korea in 2015, that was started by a person who had just returned from the Arabian peninsula. So far, all cases have been caused by visits to, or residence in, that region. MERS is zoonotic, its reservoir being in camels, which snort droplets into the air, and should be avoided, despite any locals hustling tourists to take camel rides. Symptoms of MERS in humans appear within a range from two to fourteen days after infection, so it is quite possible to fly home after a business trip to the Middle East, unknowingly carrying MERS, as has happened with travellers returning to Algeria, Austria, China, Egypt, France, Germany, Greece, Italy, Korea, Malaysia, Netherlands, Philippines, Thailand, Tunisia, Turkey, United Kingdom and United States of America. Although identified in September 2012, MERS continues to cause sporadic and localised outbreaks.

Some infected people have mild symptoms, like a common cold, but most suffer distressing respiratory symptoms causing 30-40 per cent fatalities, the majority of which occur in patients with a pre-existing medical condition that weakened their immune system, such as diabetes, cancer, chronic lung disease, heart disease or kidney disease. More severe symptoms include fever, coughing and shortness of breath, sometimes nausea, diarrhoea and vomiting – and, for some, more severe complications, such as pneumonia and kidney failure. This virus is highly infectious, attacking nursing and medical staff and people living with an infected person through droplets expelled when the sufferer coughs. There is, at the time of writing, no vaccine for MERS. Youth and age are no defence: victims' ages range from less than 1 year old to 99 years old.

WHO is concerned that this highly virulent pathogen could become a pandemic, and monitors every reported outbreak with CDC, which issues guidance for travellers to the Middle East and informs health services and hospitals in many countries of the risks associated with MERS. However, we remember the situation in mid-December 2019 when patients were already suffering and dying in Wuhan of respiratory problems and high fevers that did not respond to conventional 'flu treatments. On 27 December the Chinese equivalent of *Financial Times* known as *Caixin* reported what the Chinese Academy of Medical Sciences already knew. As it happened, the Wuhan-based virologist who had traced the vector of SARS virus to infected bats living in a cave, Shi Zhengli, was attending a conference in Shanghai. Seeing the *Caixin article,* she immediately headed back to Wuhan at the same time as Gao Fu, director of the Chinese Centre for Control and Prevention of Disease despatched a team of his virologists there.

On 31 December Dr Michael Ryan, the WHO chief of emergencies, learned about the outbreak for the first time. On 1 January WHO requested information from its contacts in China. Within the mandatory forty-eight hours, they reported forty-eight cases and no deaths. Shi Zhengli did not waste time, but published the entire genome of the coronavirus on 2 January. WHO director general Tedros Ghebreyesus later said China had set a new standard for outbreak response, but on 3 January *Caixin* reported that the Chinese health authorities had issued a confidential instruction for all samples of the virus to be destroyed or sent into safe keeping, and forbade any institute to publish any news about its findings. This applied also to Shi Jengli's laboratory.

On 5 January WHO announced 'an unusual cluster of pneumonia cases with no fatalities in Wuhan'. Chinese virologist Zhang Yongzhen had succeeded in sequencing the virus and informed the international GenBank database of virus sequences, warning the new virus was similar to SARS and 'likely infectious' and notifying the Chinese National Health Commission that he had done so. WHO, however, considered that there was no evidence of transmission between human victims and failed to recommend any specific measures for travellers. In China's CDC laboratory, technicians prepared testing guidelines and devised testing kits, although this urgent measure was confidential to those directly involved and not communicated to all staff. For two weeks, the official word from Wuhan was that there were no new cases. Researchers, however, had found that the still unnamed virus could bind itself to human cells.

On 7 January 2020 a team of specialists in Wuhan announced that they had sequenced the novel coronavirus, confirming Shi Zhengli's findings. The Associated Press news site reported that the Chinese CDC announced they 'did not trust her findings and needed to verify her data before she could publish'. AP added that the CDC was trying to prevent publication of Shi's work so they could publish first. A coronavirus researcher at University of Pennsylvania said it was a matter of 'face' in that the CDC wanted to take all the credit. By now, even some CDC staff members were wondering why it was taking so long to officially identify the novel coronavirus.

On 8 January 2020 the *Wall Street Journal* reported a novel coronavirus had been identified in samples from pneumonia patients in Wuhan. The article was profoundly embarrassing to the Chinese authorities. Later, even lab technicians in Wuhan admitted that the first they heard about the novel coronavirus was the story in the *Wall Street Journal* because their own government was still denying the nature of the new coronavirus more than a week after three Chinese medical laboratories had independently decoded the information. Other nations, including the US with its enormous intelligence-gathering community, showed no alarm. The World Health Organisation congratulated China for its rapid sequencing of the novel virus and sharing the information internationally, despite it having concealed that information. So was anyone actually 'keeping track' of the outbreak? Dr Tom Grein, chief of the World Health Organisation's acute management team, went on record as saying afterwards that WHO looked 'doubly, incredibly stupid' [for failing to denounce the lack of transparency in Beijing]. The fact is we're two to three weeks into an event. We don't have a laboratory diagnosis, we don't have an age, sex or geographic distribution, we don't have an epidemic curve [a graphic of outbreaks used to indicate the progress of an epidemic].' The problem for all international agencies is that they recoil from denouncing any member state, and China is a member of WHO, as are all UN members except Liechtenstein.

The editors of *The New England Journal of Medicine* know their business, and launched an informed outcry in the issue of 8 October 2020:

> Covid-19 has created a crisis throughout the world. Our leaders have taken a crisis and turned it into a tragedy. The United States leads the world in Covid-19 cases and in deaths due to the disease. The death rate in this country is more than double that of Canada, exceeds that of Japan by a factor of almost 50, and even dwarfs the rates in countries such as Vietnam, by a factor of almost 2,000.
>
> China chose strict quarantine and isolation after an initial delay, reducing the death rate to a reported 3 per million, as compared with more than 500 per million in the United States. Singapore and South Korea began intensive testing early, and have had relatively small outbreaks. Not only have many democracies done better than the United States, but they have also outperformed us by orders of magnitude.
>
> When the disease first arrived, we were incapable of testing effectively and couldn't provide even the most basic personal protective equipment to health care workers. The number of tests performed per infected person puts us far below such places as Kazakhstan, Zimbabwe, and Ethiopia. In much of the [US], people simply don't wear masks, largely because our leaders have stated outright that masks are political tools rather than effective infection control measures.

The United States came into this crisis with enormous advantages [including] a biomedical research system that is the envy of the world. Yet, instead of relying on expertise, the administration has obscure[d] the truth and facilitate[d] the promulgation of outright lies. More than 200,000 Americans have died.

When it comes to the response to the largest public health crisis of our time, our current political leaders have demonstrated that they are dangerously incompetent.

We should not abet the deaths of thousands more Americans by allowing [those leaders] to keep their jobs.[3]

In London, the conduct of Prime Minister Boris Johnson and his government had not been much more effective that than of the Trump administration in Washington. Johnson himself pooh-pooed the danger of Covid-19 until he caught it and was rushed into intensive care at St Thomas' Hospital in April 2020. Every day that year a visually impressively staged press conference carried on British TV channels purported to give the current state of the pandemic as it affected Britain, but the performance was long on promises and very short on achievement. Perhaps lying on television about a serious problem facing the entire nation is tiring for a politician. Either for this reason or some other, just about every member of Johnson's cabinet became the 'expert for a day' sooner or later. When a medically qualified person was interviewed on television, the gushing praise for the government's 'achievements' was notably missing.

Meanwhile, research laboratories, both state-funded and in the pharmacological industries of many developed countries, were working flat out to try and find a vaccine. To distract attention from his own ill-informed announcements during the pandemic, US President Trump accused WHO of colluding with Beijing. In fact, the WHO had been fed by China only the minimal information required by international law. Later, staff members of WHO hinted that their strategy had been to stay as China-friendly as possible in the hope of gradually prising more information from reluctant officials in Beijing. Despite the Chinese CDC being pushed by the *Wall Street Journal* article to officially announce the discovery of the new coronavirus, it still did not release the genome of the virus; it failed to make public any diagnostic tests or data that would show how infectious the virus was.

Alert immigration officers in Thailand isolated a female passenger from Wuhan with a runny nose, sore throat and high temperature. Professor Supaporn Wacharapluesadee from Chulalongkorn University in Bangkok examined the passenger and pronounced her infected with a new coronavirus, very similar to what Chinese officials had described. The professor and her team at the university independently worked out the genetic sequence by 9 January and reported the findings to the Thai government.

On 19 March 2020 it was announced in New York that the Chinese ultra-hi-tech lab start-up company Vision Medicals, based at Guangzhou in Guangdong Province had completed its clinical sequencing assay of SARS CoV-2, aka Covid-19, using next-generation sequencing. For readers able to understand the technical terms, the test was built on a proprietary metagenomic sequencing assay that runs on an Illumina NextSeq sequencer. Each kit contains thirty-eight tests and is able to detect SARS-CoV-2 at a sensitivity of 500 copies per milliliter.

Wuhan (population 11.08 million) is the chief city in the Central Chinese province of Hubei. On 1 January 2020 Dr Ai Fen, working in a Wuhan hospital reported on a Chinese social media platform that she and her colleagues were fighting a strange form of pneumonia. For her pains, she was reprimanded by the hospital's disciplinary committee for spreading unsubstantiated rumours and eight of her colleagues were arrested by the Wuhan Public Security Bureau (PSB) for the same offence. In the battle of initials, the PSB found itself opposing WHO, which announced that it was on an emergency footing to deal with a potentially serious epidemic. The PSB shut down a seafood market in Wuhan, where the health authorities forbade medical staff from speaking or writing about the new virus. They maintained that there had been no person-to-person transmission of the new pneumonia. On 7 January Chinese President Xi Jinping discussed the new disease in the Politburo. On 8 January the Chinese Health Ministry announced that the new pneumonia epidemic was caused by a novel coronavirus related to SARS and MERS, and published its genome, enabling scientists in other countries to begin developing tests for the virus.

This was timely because on 8 January WHO reported the first case of the pneumonia outside China – in a traveller returning to Thailand from Wuhan. In Hubei province all was officially imposed silence while the annual congress of the Communist Party took place, but on 14 January unofficial reports leaked out from Wuhan hospitals that suggested only person-to-person transmission could have produced the flood of new cases in the city. On the following day, WHAM! A traveller from Wuhan was diagnosed with the infection in the USA. On 20 January, the news was official: person-to-person contagion was confirmed by China's National Health Commission and the Republic of South Korea announced its first case. An official WHO delegation visiting Wuhan was inconclusive.

People's Daily, the Chinese national newspaper used the word *coronavirus* for the first time on 21 January. There were officially 291 cases, but the message was that President Xi was going to sort it all out. So, nothing to worry about ... In Beijing the municipal government declared that anyone covering up the outbreak 'will be nailed on the pillar of shame for eternity'. That was some turn-around in just seven days! WHO could not decide whether to declare Covid-19 a potential pandemic. Nobody in Wuhan was under any illusions when the entire city was placed under lockdown, isolated from the rest of the country. Not wishing to alienate an important member state, WHO decided not to declare a global emergency yet. By 23 January more than 400 people were infected and seventeen had died.

Millions of Chinese travelled across the vast country to celebrate the Chinese Lunar New Year with families in the week of 24–30 January, but there was no holiday for thousands of construction workers drafted in to build and equip *fast*, working against the clock, two entirely new hospitals in Wuhan, to cope with the flood of new cases. On 26 January the central government in Beijing imposed a nationwide ban on the trade in wild animals for food. On 28 January, with eighty-two confirmed cases outside China, Dr Tedros Ghebreyesus, director general of WHO, met President Xi to advise him that WHO must declare that Covid-19 was turning into a global pandemic. The cat – or, rather, the virus – was finally out of the bag. At first, it was thought that the locals were catching the new coronavirus after eating pangolins bought in so-called wet markets, where customers buy living animals, which are either killed, skinned and butchered at the time of purchase by the stallholder or taken away alive and killed by the customer at home.

Despite its reptilian appearance, the pangolin is a mammal, with long, sharp claws it uses for digging out ants to eat and hard overlapping protective scales covering its whole body. It has, however, no instinct to use those claws to defend itself against predators. When threatened, it just curls up into a ball, making it very easy for hunters to pick up and stuff into a cage or basket in defiance of the Chinese law that penalises people selling pangolins with up to ten years' imprisonment.

Thanks to the illegal traffic, millions are caught and eaten every year as adults and even foetuses, mostly in Asia and Africa, driving the species to extinction according to Sir David Attenbrough. Rather like skunks, pangolins secrete an unpleasant odour from glands near the anus, using this to mark their territory. After cooking, this odour also permeates the meat on the table. So why eat it? According to traditional Chinese medicine, parts of the animal have medicinal properties, although this is as unproven as the belief which sees hundreds of rhinoceroses killed by poachers each year because powdered rhino horn is believed by millions of anxious Asian men that it will remedy their erectile dysfunction.

Not just the pangolin's flesh, but also its scales, are used. When dried, they are roasted to ashes, crushed to powder, cooked with butter, vinegar and oil, plus boys' urine! Sometimes they are compressed into pills or mixed with sieved earth or crushed oyster shells, diluting the 'medicine' and making more money for the dealer. Used as medicine, this magic powder is supposed to cure problems with breast-feeding, also skin diseases, dysmenorrhoea and arthritis. Some Africans also believe that eating the meat cures kidney problems, despite there being no evidence of this either. However, the first apparent explanation of Covid-19 was that it infected people who ate pangolin meat improperly cooked, allowing the unkilled pathogen to infect them, after which they infected others.

If all that is like something from the remote past, there is also, just outside the city of Wuhan, the Wuhan Institute of Virology, an ultra-secure biosafety Level 4 laboratory opened in 2015. The institute has a suspected germ warfare role, if one believes former US President Trump and Vice-President Mike Pence, despite American intelligence agencies not agreeing with them. According to the president, Wuhan suffered the first outbreak because some of the pathogen escaped from WIV, due to poor laboratory hygiene, as when SARS virus twice escaped from a lab in Beijing in 2004. On 27 April of that year, Associated Press (AP) news agency carried this article:

> Bob Dietz, WHO spokesman in Beijing, told us on Monday (April 26) that the latest outbreak of severe acute respiratory

syndrome (SARS) in China, with eight confirmed or suspected cases so far and hundreds quarantined, involves two researchers who were working with the virus in a Beijing research lab. 'We suspect two people,' he said, 'A 26-year-old female postgraduate student and a 31-year-old male postdoc lab worker, were both infected, apparently in two separate incidents.'

The woman was admitted to hospital on April 4, but the man apparently became infected independently two weeks later, being hospitalized on April 17. Both worked at the Chinese Institute of Virology in Beijing, part of China's Center for Disease Control.

At a news conference in Manila this morning, WHO Western Pacific Regional Director Shigeru Omi criticized that laboratory's safeguards and said the authorities did not know yet whether any foreigners had been carrying out medical research in the facility and had since left the country. Laboratory safety 'is a serious issue that has to be addressed', he said. 'We have to remain very vigilant. China has Level 3 research guidelines and rules in place for handling the SARS virus, which are of acceptable quality to WHO, but it's a question of procedures and equipment. Frankly we are going to go in now a take a very close look.'

'We have a team of two or three international experts that's arriving [there] in a day or two,' Dietz said. 'They are going to go into the labs with Ministry of Health people and find out what happened here. We've been told we'll have full access, be able to test all the surfaces, interview people who worked there, and look at documentation to find out what was being done. We're not releasing the names of the experts yet, but once you see the names you'll recognize them. They will be international experts from the relevant disciplines.'

In the meantime, the lab has been closed, and the 200 staff [members] have been put in isolation in a hotel near another lab in Cham Ping, about 20 kilometers north of Beijing. China is rushing its own investigative teams to check lab security, according to state media.

Antoine Danchin, an epidemiologist with the Hong Kong University-Pasteur Research Center, who studied the SARS epidemic in Hong Kong, told [AP that] the latest incidents were probably the result of lab accidents. 'Normally, it's not possible to contaminate people even under level two confinement, if the security rules are obeyed, with the appropriate hoods, and so on,' he said. 'SARS work requires Level 3 security [which] suggests there has been some mishandling of something. The lab might have all the right rules, but the people may not comply! For example, notebooks are not supposed to be taken out, a lot of things like that. A virus doesn't jump on people!'

However WHO Beijing is relatively sanguine about the current threat, despite the fact that the 26-year-old female [postgraduate lab worker] had taken a long journey on the country's rail network while infected.[4]

That incident led President Trump at one point to suggest that the novel coronavirus had been deliberately 'leaked' from the Wuhan lab in a biological warfare operation. Western virologists found the conspiracy theories unlikely, pointing out that up to 7 million people in Southeast Asia are infected with bat coronaviruses each year. And yet ... mystery surrounds the WIV, not least because two of its researchers – Keding Ching and his wife Xiangguo Qiu – were working in Canada's National Microbiology Laboratory until expelled in 2019 for unspecified breaches of security.

Previously, staff at WIV came into the news in 2005, when they published a five-year research programme indicating that cave-dwelling Chinese horseshoe bats are a natural reservoir for coronaviruses. In 2017 the WIV hypothesised that coronaviruses found in these bats in Yunnan province could be the origin of human SARS virus. A year later, they reported that some people living near the bat caves had antibodies indicating that they had been infected by the bat coronaviruses. At the end of 2019 an outbreak of viral pneumonia was said to have been caused by a virus similar to the RaTG13 virus in those bats.

Within two weeks NIAID researchers were able to describe how the coronaviruses enter human cells using their protein spikes to 'unlock' the cells' natural defences. Once inside, they can delay the body's immune system responses to invasion until they are firmly established. Within two months various drug companies were conducting trials of possible cures and vaccines. The National Institute of Allergy and Infectious Diseases, headquartered in Maryland, USA, conducting tests on various monkey and mice species of lab animals at its Rocky Mountain Laboratory (RML) in Montana demonstrated that MERS is detectable medically within twenty-four hours of infection, causing pneumonia deep within the lungs making the victim shed virus-laden droplets from nose and throat. Not surprisingly, sufferers with pre-existing conditions like diabetes, hypertension, cardiovascular problems, cancer, obesity, respiratory problems, chromosomal defects and chronic kidney disease are particularly at risk, as are small infants and the elderly.

Chapter 14

Pandemic and Panic

The emergence of SARS-CoV2 , aka Covid-19, in December 2019, was declared a global pandemic by WHO on 11 March 2020. How did it spread so far, so fast?

In 2020 many sports fans resented the ban on attending matches during the coronavirus quarantine. Spectators cheering their team and ecstatically hugging and kissing fellow supporters after a goal release billions of droplets of infection into the air, as happened when 40,000 fans crowded into the San Siro stadium in Milan on 19 February 2010 for a Champions League football match between the Bergamo team Atalanta and the Valencia team, who brought 2,500 fans with them from Spain, This was two days before Covid-19 was first diagnosed in Italy. 'But on the day,' declared Bergamo mayor Giorgio Gori, 'no one knew the virus was already here.'

They would soon find out. Within three weeks of the match, Northern Italy had the highest number of Covid-19 infections and deaths in the entire world, apart from China. But the virus did not stop there. Sports fans travel all over the world to see a match. In this case, they took back with them not just memories, but also Covid-19. Track-and-trace on people who travelled back home after the fatal match show that, in Africa, they brought the infection with them to Algeria, Central African Republic, Côte d'Ivoire, Morocco, Nigeria, Senegal, the Seychelles, South Africa and Tunisia. In football-mad Latin America and the Caribbean, the virus reached Argentina, Bolivia, Brazil, Chile, Colombia, Cuba, Dominican Republic, Guatemala, Mexico, Uruguay and Venezuela. In Asia, India, Bangladesh, China, Malaysia, the Maldives, Japan all got a dose of Milanese Covid. In North America, cases in the United States and Canada were traced back to Milan. In the Middle East other cases traced back to the match appeared in Israel, Jordan, Oman, Saudi Arabia, United Arab Emirates. In Asia, fans took the virus back to South Korea, Sri Lanka, Thailand, Vietnam. European fans brought it back to Albania, Andorra, Austria, Belgium, Belarus, Bosnia-Herzegovina, Croatia, Cyprus, Czech Republic, Denmark, Estonia, Finland, France, Germany, Greece, Hungary, Ireland, Iceland, Latvia, Lithuania, Luxemburg, Malta, Moldova, Netherlands, North Makedonia, Norway, Poland, Portugal, Romania, San Marino, Serbia, Slovakia, Slovenia, Spain, Sweden, Switzerland, Ukraine and the United Kingdom. In the former USSR, fans who had been present at the match in Milan also took the virus back with them to Armenia, Azerbaijan, Georgia and Russia. There was even one woman who returned from Northern Italy to New Zealand with the bug, and was diagnosed in Auckland on 4 March 2020.

Cheap air travel was going to claim thousands of lives in the next few months: a geometric progression from the 12,000 people who died of Spanish 'flu in 1918 after attending the street parade in Philadelphia. In the first year of Covid-19, disinterested observers have commented how the three and a half centuries since 1666–67, which have produced 90 per cent of all scientific knowledge, have provided no new tools to stop a pandemic spreading than were available in Pepys' London. Isolation, at times and in many places observed only casually, was the only measure available, it seemed, until a vaccine was invented. Prime Minister Boris Johnson himself pooh-pooed the danger of Covid-19 until he caught it and was rushed into intensive care at St Thomas' Hospital in April 2020. Every day a high profile staged press conference carried on British TV channels purported to give the current state of events, but the performance was long on promises and very short on achievement. Perhaps lying on television about a serious problem facing the entire nation is tiring for a politician. Either for this reason or some other, just about every member of Johnson's cabinet became the 'expert for a day' sooner or later, although when a medically qualified person was interviewed on television, any gushing praise for the government's 'achievements' was notably missing.

Meanwhile, research laboratories, both state-funded and in the pharmacological industries of many developed countries, were working flat out to try and find a vaccine, which proved as elusive as the Holy Grail.

In May 2020 the PSB arrested a 37-year-old 'citizen-journalist' named Zhang Zhan for putting on social media news about what was happening in Wuhan. Seven or eight others were also arrested for the same 'crime'. She was not tried until November, when her sentence was four years' imprisonment for disturbing public order. Her lawyer courageously told the world that she considered herself innocent, was on a prolonged hunger strike in protest at her detention and was being forcibly fed in prison; he feared that she might die. According to the Committee to Protect Journalists, based in New York, also still in jail were fellow protesters Chen Qiushi and Fang Bin. Once again, the Chinese government had showed the world how far it was willing to go, to suppress awkward truths.

On 29 December 2020 BBC News reminded the world of Dr Li Wenliang, who died on 7 February, accused of 'disturbing social order' and 'making false comments' for warning colleagues about Covid-19. More than 1 million courageous Chinese posted on Sina Weibo social media messages of support for his memory – messages that were regularly wiped by the authorities. A journalist named Li Zehua posted a You tube video in February of himself being chased in a car by police. He then disappeared for two months, surfacing to say that he had been 'cooperating with the authorities'. A Wuhan author named Fang Fang, who wrote an online diary documenting her life in the city, cut off from the rest of China, was accused of smearing China's good name.

BBC News on 30 December 2020 reported that researchers at the Chinese CDC found that 5 per cent of people in Wuhan had been infected by Covid-19. That works out at half a million people, almost ten times higher than the official figure of 50,354.

By the end of 2020 Covid-19 had claimed 1.8 million lives worldwide, but it seemed at last that the end of the pandemic was in sight as competing Big Pharma companies in America, Europe and Russia all announced at pretty much the same time that they were on the verge of marketing their different vaccines, each of which was claimed to have 90 or 95 per cent efficacy against the coronavirus. There was inevitably some foot-dragging on the part of the Food and Drugs Administration in the USA and other government approval bodies in Europe, rightly concerned that many people might have allergic reactions to the vaccines. It did not seem that President Putin's Russia was too worried about the safety of its vaccine: what did a few thousand allergic reactions matter in the population of the twenty-two republics of the Russian Federation, totalling 146 million people?

But then! In December the New and Emerging Respiratory Virus Threats Advisory Group (NERVTAG) announced that Covid-19 had mutated in southeast England. The Group's chairman, Professor Peter Horby told the House of Commons Science and Technology Committee that the variant designated 501.v2 appeared to have originated in one person in Kent. Seventy per cent more contagious, it was spreading much more rapidly than the other versions.

Bad news? Worse was to come.

The new variant had been detected on 21 September but Nervtag and Public Health England had learned of it just a fortnight previously. Why the delay? Almost at the same time, just before Christmas, Professor Lawrence Young, a molecular oncologist at Warwick Medical School, announced that another variant was rampaging through the Eastern and Western Cape states of the Union of South Africa, and had arrived in Britain, brought by two travellers returning from South Africa. It was as if the virus was defending itself from the imminent vaccine attack. Of course, an individual virus has no brain as such, but when we watch a flock of hundreds of birds flying in tight formation executing split-second manouvres without any mid-air collisions, we have to wonder how they are communicating. A school of thousands of fish can likewise take co-ordinated evading action from an approaching shark at similar speed with, again, no collisions. How do they do it? We don't know, but if they had not been doing this for thousands of years, their marine predators would have wiped them out. The globe-shaped nests of Asian hornets hanging in our trees require a group intelligence as architect and the collaboration of the whole community in the construction. Honeybees coordinate their pollen gathering and take group decisions about creating a new community. Although each hive or nest has a queen, her role is simply to create more worker bees, so she takes no part in the group decisions, which happen in some way democratically by a majority vote. Ants also co-ordinate their activities.

People began to wonder whether the billions or trillions of Covid-19 viruses were together capable of working out the time to mutate in the face of the imminently available vaccines. Not so. Professor Young explained that variants of Covid-19 had been around since the beginning of the pandemic. It was, he said, a normal way in which a virus developed and adapted to its hosts when replicating in them. But, if the mutations were random, one would expect a roughly equal number of mutations weakening the viruses as the ones improving their ability to infect and making them more resistant to the human immune response. But that is not so, leaving one to wonder what intelligence is driving the mutations. In the case of Covid-19, already in April 2020 doctors in Sweden found that it had developed two genetic changes, which made it twice as infectious. By the end of the year *many thousands of the mutations* had been identified around the world.

No sooner had the existence of vaccines been announced than low-cost Ryanair came up with the slogan *Jab and Go!* Business is business, but it seemed socially irresponsible in the midst of a severe new peak of infections, with the huge Nightingale emergency hospitals manned by army personnel on alert for a new wave of coronavirus victims, to encourage the public to even think of flying from country to country for business or pleasure.

Chapter 15

Pathogens A-plenty

The smallpox doctor Edward Jenner wrote more than two centuries ago, in 1798:

> The deviation of man from the state in which he was placed by nature seems to have proved to him a prolific source of diseases

The WHO announced on 8 May 1980 that smallpox had been eradicated from the entire planet – except, of course, for the stockpiles retained in military laboratories of many countries. The USSR at the time had twenty tons of *variola major* viruses stored in Zagorsk.[1] Given the weight of a single virus, that's enough to kill the entire human race.

Right now, several sub-Saharan countries are experiencing a plague of locusts, producing starvation for millions and a suitable breeding ground for a new epidemic. And then there are viruses that attack farm animals in reasonably natural conditions – among them, anthrax, fowl pest, swine fever and foot-and-mouth disease, any one of which may jump species to us. Krausfeldt-Jacob disease in humans is thought to come from cattle infected with bovine spongiform encephalopathy – commonly called mad cow disease. Due to factory farming and the consequent 'necessity' to treat with antibiotics animals and fowl reared under the deeply unnatural intensive conditions, in 1961 a new disease was diagnosed in British hospitals: MRSA or methicillin-resistant staphylococcus aureus. A variant acquired in normal life and not in hospitals, known as CA-MRSA also now exists. Treatable by newly developed antibiotics if caught at the right moment, CA-MRSA has all the potential to become epidemic, defying available medical treatment. Every winter up to 500,000 ordinary 'flu sufferers die, but in developed countries annual anti-flu jabs give a good degree of immunity, *so far.* But when a variant like H5N1 – the avian 'flu of 2003 or the Hong Kong 'flu H3N2 of 1968–70 appears, millions die.

On 16 November 2020 the PBS satellite channel broadcast a programme under the title *The Virus: What Went Wrong?* In it, respected journalist Martin Smith took viewers through all the relevant events from 17 November 2019, when the first announcement was made to several colleagues by a doctor in Wuhan about the new coronavirus causing temperatures as high as 42 degrees Centigrade (105 degrees Fahrenheit) and severe respiratory problems, i.e. fatal pneumonia. The Chinese Public Security Bureau – an all-powerful agency for the suppression of news and activities considered undesirable by the government of China – ordered the doctor responsible to cease and desist under threat of instant arrest if he repeated the 'offence'. He escaped that threat by dying in intensive care from infection by Covid-19. Meanwhile, research revealed that the genome of Covid-19 was 80 per cent the same as that of SARS, but the difference was such that the same drugs would not work with Covid-19.

On 20 January WHO repeated the Chinese 'party line' that there was no person-to-person transmission. The lunar New Year began on 25 January, with millions of Chinese having travelled all across China to spend the annual celebrations with their families. Too late, the authorities in Wuhan isolated the entire city of 11.08 million inhabitants, or rather those that remained; the others were spreading the virus all over the country. According to Chinese-American researcher Dr David Ho, the reason why no warning was made about the danger by the government in Beijing was the tradition that giving bad news during the New Year period would cause bad happenings to the person giving the news! The Romans had a more appropriate saying: *si pacem vis, para bellum* – if you want peace, prepare for war. Whether US President Barak Obama studied Latin at school is unknown, although he did once have a name-plate carrying the words *Vero possemus* – Latin for his campaign slogan *Yes we can*. Latinist or not, he realised that anti-epidemic precautions need to be in place *before* the next one comes, and therefore set up *inside* the White House the Pandemic Response Unit. His successor, President Donald Trump had decided this was unnecessary and banished the weakened response unit to another building, where it lacked the authority given by Obama. There was thus no prior response before people started dying in the USA in increasing numbers, and not then either. On 26 February Trump informed the American public that the US was the best prepared country in the world. He also denied the infectiousness of the novel coronavirus even after he caught it and was hospitalised. Or did he really catch it? He was famous for so many lies during his presidency that it is quite possible he only pretended to have the virus so he could say it was no worse than seasonal 'flu.

Meanwhile, back in London Prime Minister Boris Johnson also scorned the danger of Covid-19 until he caught it and was rushed into intensive care in hospital. Britain was similarly unprepared and its government also procrastinated until introducing quarantine restrictions – terming them *lockdowns*, an expression used in American penitentiaries for forcing recalcitrant prisoners back into their cells after a riot. But a lockdown of 124 days did not stop the virus, instead doing terrible damage to the UK economy. Therein lies the dilemma: will future political leaders prepare for pandemics or simply prepare alibis while prioritising economic issues?

And what about that endemic disease of the nineteenth century, then called 'consumption'? The author's father died of its consequences despite the best treatment available in early-50s Britain. If now very rare in Europe, tuberculosis is alive and thriving in Asia. Unbeknown to the Western tourists who stroll through an Indian bazaar or street market, one third of the gaily dressed natives around them are infected with it, even if not visibly manifesting the disease. Although today a cure is available for those with the money to buy three or four different drugs and take them daily for a period of six to eight months, the Asian sufferer's money often runs out part-way through the course. This creates a drug-resistant variant of the TB bacillus *mycobacterium tuberculosis*, even more difficult for doctors to cure because 70 per cent of the TB strains isolated are now resistant to the drugs that used to cure this disease.[2] It may surprise readers to learn that WHO predicts that deaths from TB currently total 2.5 million per annum and are likely to rise soon to 3.5 million.[3]

Across the world in eastern Peru the local epidemiologist in the remote Amazonian jungle town of Iquitos is accustomed to finding in every village she visits, however small, one or two people who cough up blood. Iquitos is the largest town in the world with no road access, but only river-boat and air links. It suffered 27,000 cases of cholera diagnosed in 1991 with 426 deaths. Persistent and very courageous itinerant health workers dropped this to 6,000 cases in 1992, 5,500 in 1993 and so on down. The main reason why this did not become an epidemic was the difficulty of access, although the local government is now trying to create a tourist trade. The worried government in Lima doubled the wages of doctors and nurses working in this remote area, which now has fifty healthcare professionals combating dozens of tropical diseases. Malaria is endemic and the cases of the more malignant *falciparum* malaria is now resistant to all but very expensive antibiotics, for which there is no money locally.

Another pathogen, carried by the bite of infected phlebotomine female sandflies is the cause of leishmaniasis, which can eat away the flesh of the face. Leprosy, although long extinct in Europe, is still common, as is fulminant hepatitis, often mistaken for yellow fever, which thrives in the area. The directory of tropical diseases in Amazonia would not be complete without mentioning histolytic amoebiasis, a vicious haemolytic disease called *verruga peruiana* and Chagas' disease.[4]

As if all these lurking threats were not enough, a number of developed countries have institutions for what they call bio-defence. The Pentagon spends $91 million per annum to develop lethal pathogens that could be used for biological warfare, using the argument that only thus can it protect the American people by creating treatments for them, necessary should these pathogens ever be turned on them by another country. Britain has the Defence Science and Technology Laboratory and other facilities at Porton Down, near Salisbury, and argues similarly, as do other European states. In the former USSR, now the Russian Federation, is a staggering stockpile of bio-warfare agents left over from the Cold War.

Long before these modern facilities, the Japanese army ran a facility in occupied Manchuria officially designated Water Purification Unit 731. Starting in the late 1930s, under Lieutenant General Shiro Ishi this unit of 3,600 specialists at Pingfang in Harbin carried out experiments exposing some 10,000 Manchurian and Chinese prisoners and some unfortunate British, Russian and American POWs to virulent strains of anthrax, dysentery, cholera and plague. As if that were not bad enough, the guinea pigs were subsequently subjected to agonising vivisection without anaesthetic to assess the effects on their internal organs. During the Sino-Japanese war (1937–45) Ishii ordered fragile porcelain containers to be air-dropped over Chinese cities, shattering on impact to release hundreds of fleas infected with plague and other weaponised pathogens. At the end of the Second World War, after Soviet troops occupied Manchuria, Japanese prisoners from Pingfang, if taken by the Soviets, were placed on trial for war crimes in Khabarovsk and the records of Unit 731 recovered with them were carted off to Moscow, including blueprints for biolabs in which the pathogens could safely be weaponised. These were used by Soviet scientists to vastly increase their own output of bio-weapons. Yet, Ishii and a few of Unit 731's top brass managed to get back to Japan and surrender themselves to American forces. In return for immunity from prosecution for war crimes in the Tokyo trials – while leaving behind in Manchuria a handful of lower-echelon operatives to be put on trial by the Soviets, for the sake of appearances – they handed over what purported to be the complete records of Unit 731. The US government apparently used this research obtained by inhumane means for experiments on jailed criminals and black citizens, the latter on the pretext that it was necessary to create special vaccines for coloured persons. During the Korean War (1950–53) it was alleged that US or South Korean aircraft dropped some of these weaponised pathogens on North Korean towns.

At the same time in the incipient Cold War between the Warsaw Pact and NATO, the Soviet Ministry of Agriculture was developing and weaponising viruses and bacteria including foot-and-mouth disease and rinderpest, glanders, swine fever and fowl pest in preparations suitable to be sprayed from low-flying aircraft. Using the pen-name Ken Alibek, an ethnic Kazakh whose real name was Kanatjan Alibekov was a former director of Stalin's Biopreparat – euphemistically translated as the Institute of Applied Biochemistry – in Omutninsk, 600 miles east of Moscow. He published a history of Biopreparat after moving to the West on the collapse of the USSR.[5]

In the West, the start of the Covid-19 panic included allegations that the virus had leaked – whether intentionally or not – from the Wuhan laboratory. These things do happen. One thousand miles northwest of Wuhan in the province of Ganso is the city of Lanzhou with the China Animal Husbandry Biopharmaceutical Laboratory, which is said to specialise in developing vaccines for the country's huge agricultural industry. In 2019, the management tried to cut costs by buying some out-of-date disinfectant. In July and August when used to treat the air vented from the facility, this failed to eliminate live brucella bacteria, which formed aerosols that floated away, hitting first the nearby

Lanzhou Veterinary Research Institute and Lanzhou University, where 200-plus people were infected, according to Xinhua news agency. A total of 3,245 people living close and a further 1,401 people in the region also tested positive for brucellosis. The local health authority said there was no evidence of person-to-person transmission – humans normally get the disease by contact with infected animals, by consuming unpasteurised milk or eating undercooked meat – but that still makes a large number of people suffering high fevers with copious sweating, headaches and joint pain. Seven out of ten would have gastrointestinal symptoms such as nausea, vomiting, low appetite, weight loss, constipation or diarrhoea, liver trouble and even an enlarged spleen. In severe cases, the central nervous system and lining of the heart may be affected. Sometimes, the effects take months to recede and they can last for life with secondary effects that include arthritis, meningitis and several neurological disorders collectively known as neurobrucellosis. The disabling effects of brucella bacilli are such that they were even weaponised in the Second World War, to be used by the US air forces in the M114 bursting bomblet originally developed for spreading anthrax.

Bio-warfare attacks can also come from some terrorist organisation. Does that sound far-fetched? In 1995 the Aum Shinrikyo cult killed eleven travellers and injured 5,500 others when unleashing the nerve gas sarin in the Tokyo subway. This is an extremely toxic organophosphorus compound, outlawed by the Chemical Weapons Convention of 1993, which produces loss of bowel and bladder control, vomiting and other symptoms, causing death in one to ten minutes after inhalation. The reason why more fatalities did not result is that the cult members making the gas in their own laboratory, transporting it to the subway and releasing it there, were amateurs. Aum Shinrikyo adherents had previously tried to carry out similar attacks using anthrax and botulinum toxin, which fortunately had failed. The Japanese terror group had sent members to Zaire during the 1992 Ebola outbreak in a failed attempt to procure samples of the Ebola virus which could be cultured in their laboratory.[6] To set up a functioning germ-warfare bio-laboratory need cost no more than £1 million, as was proven in a clandestine operation by the CIA on American soil, which the FBI never even noticed. This sum is well within the budget of several terrorist organisations subsidised by patrons in the petrochemical countries.

Our knowledge of the planet we inhabit is still largely limited to what is called the biosphere extending from just below the surface of ground or water to the upper edge of the breathable atmosphere, but US scientists have found, 870 feet below the seafloor off the Pacific Northwest coastline, microbes that were thriving there, apparently getting their energy from the chemical reaction of the rocks and sea water. In April 2020, when the human race was stunned by the novel coronavirus outbreak labelled Covid-19, professional biologists read in that month's *Communications Biology* a report by Japanese geoscientist Yohey Suzuki of thriving swarms of microbes under ancient rocks on the very bed of the South Pacific. Nobody is yet saying that these simple life-forms are dangerous to man because, so far, we have had no contact with them.

Chapter 16

A Pause for Thought

In his book *The Life of Reason*[1] the Spanish-born philosopher Jorge Augustín Nicolás Ruiz de Santayana y Borrás, later known in English as George Santayana, wrote, 'Those who cannot remember the past are condemned to repeat it.' Winston Churchill, who had a feeling for pithy sentences, borrowed this, whether knowingly or not, in a 1948 speech in the House of Commons, changing 'remember the past' to 'fail to remember history'. There is some dispute about the wording, but the meaning is clear.

Whether the Chinese Communist leader Mao Tse-Tung ever read either quote, we do not know, but he did apply the logic with his 'one-child policy' proclaimed in 1979. From an average five births per woman in China with no contraception, the result of the new policy reduced most families to two parents and one child. University graduates could have an additional child, two if both parents were graduates. Mao's policy is estimated to have prevented 400 million births. There was some cheating in rural areas, with first-born girls being clandestinely done away with, so that the parents could maybe have a son instead to help with agricultural work. How many did, is unknown, but all one-child families received a 'one-child glory certificate' for obeying, or seeming to obey, the great leader's law.

Where else and when could such a policy have been even thought of? Come to that, since he never needed to explain himself, who can say exactly what was in Mao's mind? He had extensive libraries in his many secret homes spread across China, but it seems unlikely, for geographical reasons and Mao's own mindset, that he would have read the writings of the highly respected and honoured English scientist James Lovelock. Born in 1919, he could not afford to go to university, to which he attributed his lack of becoming overspecialised in one scientific discipline.

In 1948 Lovelock received a doctorate of medicine at the London school of Hygiene and Tropical Medicine, and conducted research

157

in the United Kingdom and at Yale and Harvard universities. He was also an inventor, whose electron capture detector enabled him to detect in the atmosphere the presence of CFCs. He partly financed his own travel aboard the research ship RRS *Shackleton* from the Arctic to the Antarctic, collecting samples from the upper atmosphere as he went. Work on the damage the CFCs were evidently causing to the ozone layer won a Nobel Prize for two other scientists in 1995.

All this personal history is leading up to Lovelock's formulation of the Gaia hypothesis, which might otherwise be taken for an example of New Age pseudo-philosophy. While working in the 1960s as a NASA consultant on the Martian atmosphere in the search of extra-terrestrial life, Lovelock asked himself the question: if there is no life on Mars, but it did once exist, how can we detect its past existence? Perhaps he was wondering whether abuse by life-forms of the red planet's atmosphere accounted for its thinning to the point where it could no longer support life.[2]

This thinking led him to consider also the considerable damage already done to Earth's atmosphere, mainly due to human activity. That in turn led him to formulate the Gaia hypothesis: that life on Earth interacted with the composition of the planet. Gaia was a spelling of the Greek name for Mother Nature, present in all primitive belief systems. Lovelock was among the first to recognise the complex effect of the biosphere on the planet that supports it, and argued that the whole planet and all the life-forms on it constitute a single, complicated but delicate, symbiosis that works until one organism or groups of them, creates entropy.

Given the arrogance of human personal consciousness, this was difficult for many people to absorb. They preferred to believe that mankind was the supreme manifestation of life on Earth. Whether or not they paid lip service to a particular creed, they acted and thought as though a deity has given them ownership and jurisdiction over all other species, and over the planet itself. The early humanist philosopher Michel Eyquem de Montaigne (1533–1592) wrote in his château just a few miles from where this chapter is being written, 'Man is certainly mad. He cannot make a worm, and yet he makes gods by the dozen.'[3]

For most people, the implications of Lovelock's hypothesis were simply too worrying, especially in 2006 when he wrote *The Revenge of Gaia: Why the Earth Is Fighting Back*.[4] With apparent reason, for they had discarded Adam and Eve as the first humans, they asked how a planet could take revenge on life-forms it had created – revenge being Lovelock's metaphor for conditions hostile to the life-form that had damaged the planet. Some scientists had the intelligence and training to understand what Lovelock was on about. Bruno Latour (b. 1947), French sociologist, philosopher, anthropologist and author, is one. At Edinburgh in his 2013 Gifford Lecture – one of a series established to discuss the relationship between theology, philosophy and science – he tackled the issue of survival of both the human race and all life on the planet. 'How many times,' he asked his audience rhetorically, 'have I been told not refer to Gaia or read the books of James Lovelock?'

Latour has named the present time as the anthropocene era, in which mankind has: cut down vast swathes of the rain forests, vital for the oxygen cycle; polluted the oceans, from which much of our food comes and on which oxygen depends; poisoned, and in many places sterilised, the very ground in which we grow the greater part of our food, even perverting for commercial reasons the natural ability of grain to act as seed for the next harvest. In the process, we have exterminated so many other animal and plant species that the present qualifies as an extinction as important as the five major extinctions shown in the fossil record. Although species have died out throughout geological time, the label 'extinction' is reserved for events when *most* life on earth has been wiped out, not once, but time and again. And Latour thinks we are at the beginning of one.

The fossil record extinctions were caused by radical climate change after colossal geothermal activity and by 'nuclear winters' caused by giant asteroids slamming into Earth and blasting thousands of tons of dust into the upper atmosphere by the force of their collision, blocking sunlight and thereby killing all vegetation and the multiple species that depended on it.

The extinction that preoccupies Latour is the ongoing planetary abuse by human activity, from which people's attention is deflected, not by religion now, but by the pursuit of wealth, the trillions spent on space travel originally for military purposes, the triviality of politics, national and international, and the pressures of the consumer society, constantly implying that we have a moral duty to incur debt just to meet household needs, to buy a new car we don't need or to purchase some other particular product of Big Business.

Meanwhile, we may be forcing the planet into saving itself. Each time we disable one of its population-control weapons – death in childbirth, leprosy, malaria, measles, mumps, poliomyelitis, tuberculosis, smallpox, yellow and dengue fever, whooping cough – the list is long, and scientists are understandably acclaimed for inventing antibiotics and other achievements – another weapon is dragged from Gaia's quiver and aimed at our species in epidemic form. Since the millennium we have had epidemics of AIDS, hepatitis A and E, dengue fever, Ebola, Nipah virus, Zika virus, cholera, yellow fever, mumps, swine 'flu, chikungunya and bubonic plague, plus MERS, SARS and Coved-19. The past tense is wrong: some of these are current. Living in the temperate zone of the Northern hemisphere, most readers of this book may be dimly aware of these epidemics/pandemics, but they are for us like fake news, swiftly forgotten. Yet for the millions involved, as for every mother whose baby is dying, they are tragic reality. In addition, Biblical plagues of locusts, climate change or simple soil exhaustion make famine an ever-present menace for millions of people precariously clinging to life.

There is the Achilles' heel of the human race. The Soviet warlord Josef Djugashvili, aka Stalin, once remarked that a single death was a tragedy, whereas a million deaths was a statistic. It takes a Stalin or a Mao to have the necessarily Olympian view and the power to act. We have, of course, the United Nations Organisation and the World Health Organisation, but they cannot change major patterns of behaviour because they function by consensus. It would take a shattering pandemic, so swift in its arrival that preventive measures cannot be put in place, to restore the balance of Nature. On past form, that may yet happen.

Generally, historians confine themselves to writing about the past. Yet, Herodotus used the Greek word *'istoria* as meaning the pursuit of knowledge by enquiry, and one thing is certain. With increasingly larger cities on every continent except Antarctica, thousands of inexperienced young people taking gap years to travel internationally for fun before going to university, hundreds of thousands of business people and holiday-makers travelling internationally by air every day, with and without children, plus the large numbers of 'adventurous' tourists heading heedlessly into biological risk areas and even backpacking and camping rough there, conditions have never been more auspicious for pathogens awaiting the right moment to launch the next pandemic. We should think of them as plagues-in-waiting. To attempt to list all of them would be impossible, because some have not yet even been identified, but even the short list below of those we know makes chilling reading.

There is a ray of hope. In the summer and autumn of 2020, small regional airports all over Europe were being used as plane parks during the embargo on international travel due to Covid-19. Their hard standing was covered by civil airliners parked nose to tail and wingtip to wingtip while banned from the skies by the worldwide travel restrictions. Boeing, Airbus and other manufacturers of civil aircraft laid off thousands of skilled employees and considered a possible resumption of normal business likely in 2025 at the earliest. Civil airlines also laid off tens of thousands of personnel. Add to that the collapse in the tourism, hospitality and catering industries worldwide and it can be seen that the crises in all these areas caused by Covid-19 may ensure that the days of easy and cheap global travel are over, which might make that novel coronavirus from Wuhan a life-saver – or, at least, a life-extender – for the human species in the end, if we learn the lesson it has given us.

Apart from a few professional epidemiologists, people don't seem to ask where all the potential pandemic pathogens come from. They are the creations of the planet earth, just as much as humans, sharks, elephants, snakes and octopuses are. Although one does not normally look to popular music for great insights, at the August 1969 Woodstock festival attended in New York State by 400,000 people the group Crosby, Stills, Nash and Young[5] sang an instant hit that included the line 'We are stardust, we are golden, we are billion-year old carbon.' Golden, maybe, but certainly every atom in and on our planet is dust that has been snared in space by terrestrial gravity and an important component of our bodies and most other things is indeed billion-year-old carbon from the cosmos.

A few years after Woodstock, the visionary chemist Lovelock and microbiologist Lynn Margulis (1938–2011) floated the concept that our planet is a complicated, self-regulating *living* entity they named Gaia after the Greek earth goddess.[6] Is that any more crazy than the idea of the third rock from the sun producing life forms as different as giant molluscs and the terrestrial, marine and flying dinosaurs, humans, fish, bacteria, viruses, seaweed, grass, trees and all the materials necessary to make smart phones and the International Space Station ? The Geological Society of London had no problem in accepting Lovelock's work in 2006, when it awarded him its prestigious Wollaston Medal for significant achievement.[7]

Biologist Christopher Wills does not put it quite like that, but he's not far off. He sees the role of plagues as keeping the numbers of our species in check, which is necessary to protect the oceans and wildernesses like rain forests and all the creatures that live in them, entire species of which mankind has been progressively exterminating, either for food in the oceans or by mass killing of terrestrial 'pests', or by simply depriving them of the environment in which they have evolved. At the same time, in the last two centuries mankind's technological progress, particularly in medicine, has outwitted many of the long-established pathogens – at least in the industrialised countries. One result is the rapidly increasing size of the human race, even in the Third World where food, and particularly water, resources are already inadequate. Each year, millions of people move out of rural areas and into the cities, escaping disease vectors like mosquitoes and sand flies and schistosomiasis-carrying water snails but increasing the likelihood of diarrhoeal diseases in shanty towns and *favelas* without adequate, or any, sanitation. Perhaps the planet still has a few nasty surprises for the most destructive species it has produced.[8]

The key word in the Gaia hypothesis is 'self-regulating'. Since life first appeared on the planet, the energy received from our star the sun has increased by as much as 30 per cent. Concerned people worry today about greenhouse gases and global warming. At various times, the planet has been both far hotter and far colder than it is today. In the geological record we can see how many seemingly permanent characteristics of our planet have changed, rapidly extinguishing some life forms that had lasted millions of years and permitting new ones to evolve. The salinity of the seas, from which all life has come, has varied greatly. Photosynthetic bacteria at the beginning of the Proterozoic period modified the atmosphere, increasing oxygen content to the levels necessary for higher forms of life. In 1892 author and poet Rudyard Kipling wrote:

> Oh, East is East and West is West
> And never the Twain shall meet

Yet we know now that even the north and south poles have swapped over more than once – although we don't know why. Even gravity is not a constant. The giant terrestrial reptiles that ruled the planet millions of years ago would collapse under their own weight in today's increased gravity that compels the largest air-breathing mammals to live in the oceans.

Although some scientists, limited by their learning, have found Lovelock's hypothesis difficult to accept, he is not alone. Among other great scientists, the Scottish geologist and naturalist James Hutton (1726–1797), Prussian polymath Alexander von Humboldt (1769–1859) and Ukrainian geochemist Vladimir I. Vernadskii (1863–1945) would have understood and applauded him. Vernadskii was among the first to recognise, in his writings, that the vital gases oxygen, carbon dioxide and nitrogen did not come in a kit at the birth of the solar system, but are the result of biological process and that even small living organisms can modify the planet's atmosphere, albeit slowly to the minds of humans with our short life-spans. American environmentalist and pioneer conservationist Aldo Leopold (1887–1948), the father of wildlife ecology, also saw the planet as a living entity, developing holistic ethics regarding mankind's treatment of the land we live on. Among his sayings are:

> A thing is right when it tends to preserve the integrity, stability and beauty of the biotic community. It is wrong when it tends otherwise.
>
> We must cease being intimidated by the argument that a right action is impossible because it does not yield maximum profits, or that a wrong action is to be condoned because it pays.
>
> We abuse land because we regard it as a commodity belonging to us. When we see land [and the life-forms on it and in the sea] as a community to which we belong, we may begin to use it with love and respect.

Love and respect? Over the last century human activity has changed the world by driving to extinction thousands of species from tiny insects to giant whales. It currently continues to render extinct *each year* as many as 10,000 species from microscopic organisms to plants and animals of all sizes. Some of these undervalued species are termed buffers because they protect us from unpleasant pathogens, so we are placing ourselves at greater risk. Published in *Nature* of 2 December 2010, Professor Felicia

Keesing of Bard College in New York State wrote, 'Biodiversity loss tends to increase pathogen transmission across a wide range of infectious disease systems.' Since her speciality is the ecology of infectious diseases, we should listen to her and to her collaborator Richard Ostfield of the Cary Institute. They have, for instance, connected the decline in opossum populations due to the destruction of their habitat by US lumber companies with the consequent rise in cases of the unpleasant Lyme disease in humans. They have also focused on West Nile virus, hantavirus and nine other species of pathogens, with similar findings.

We don't have to be long-haired, bearded hippies living in cabins deep in the woods to see that from James Hutton to Leopold and Lovelock, scientifically educated thinkers of great intellect not afraid to grapple with planet-size ideas have been telling us the same or similar messages – messages that have largely gone unheeded as we continue the destruction of the vital rainforests for short-term financial gain, likewise the poisoning of the soil in which we grow our food and the contamination and pollution of the oceans, source of all life. From that, perhaps Olympian, viewpoint it can be appreciated that pandemic-producing bacteria and viruses are functioning as the planet's tools to cull the dangerous human species seemingly intent on destroying the environment that supports all life-forms.

Appendix

Below is a short list of other infections that could turn into pandemics. One of them already has.

Acquired immune deficiency syndrome (AIDS) is another scourge that emerged from African primates and 'jumped' to humans who hunted, killed and ate chimpanzees infected with simian immunodeficiency virus (SIV) without cooking the meat sufficiently to kill the virus. Or perhaps they simply came into contact with the chimps' blood while slaughtering and butchering them? The danger was first noted in the late nineteenth century, but became a potential pandemic on 5 June 1981 when a Morbidity and Mortality Weekly Report from the US CDC described five cases of *pneumonia carinii* (PCP) among previously healthy young gay men in Los Angeles, of whom two had already died. It was, of course, not the pneumonia that took their lives – although that was the immediate cause of death – but a retrovirus dubbed human immunodeficiency virus (HIV-1).

A month later, on 3 July *New York Times* carried a report that doctors in New York and California had diagnosed in New York and the San Francisco Bay area in California forty-one cases among gay men of a rare and potentially fatal form of cancer called Kaposi's sarcoma. The link was, of course, that all the men had been infected with HIV, which attacks the immune system, leaving the body unable to fight off infection and therefore vulnerable to any other disease *and to lethal cancers*.

Before the current pandemic of AIDS, some preserved blood samples, including one taken from a young man who died in northeast England during 1959, showed traces of HIV, as did tissues preserved in the port-city of Liverpool from sailors who died there years before the recognition of AIDS. So maybe it has been intermittently around for longer than was at first thought. To complicate this summary of the AIDS pandemic, there is another form of HIV, designated HIV-2, rampant in West Africa and first identified by virologists there in 1985.[1]

In the following year, the US CDC reported that more deaths from AIDS (HIV-1) were recorded for 1985 than for all previous years. The increase of 89 per cent over 1984 was fatal for 50 per cent of adult sufferers and 60 per cent of children. The world had a new pandemic, claiming between 75 and 100 million victims. Despite new drugs and treatments, in 2017 AIDS was causing the death of nearly 1 million people a year, 50 per cent more than were then dying from malaria. In some countries of sub-Saharan Africa like South Africa, Botswana and Mozambique it was the largest single cause of death. One important factor in the rapid spread of AIDS across Africa is the refusal of the Catholic Church to countenance the use of condoms.

Many heterosexual people dismiss AIDS as a disease they cannot get because the HIV virus is fragile and is only passed on in blood-to-blood contact. Yet, many women with bisexual partners have acquired this condition, to which they are especially prone if indulging in anal intercourse, the protective mucous membrane of the anus being more fragile than that of the vagina. Those women can then pass the HIV virus on to other, heterosexual, partners, as is the case with prostitutes who 'work bareback', i.e. unprotected. In Africa, where the predominant strain is HIV-2, women are particularly vulnerable if their menfolk tend not to 'waste time' on foreplay and insist on copulating *per vaginam* before the woman is physically ready, causing her to bleed during intercourse. In a number of countries on that continent public health authorities have mounted poster campaigns imploring men to accept that FOREPLAY IS IMPORTANT. Yet WHO estimates new cases of AIDS, transmitted heterosexually in Africa and Asia, at somewhere between 2 and 4 million each year.[2] HIV can also have a very long incubation period of ten years, so that intercourse with an infected partner exhibiting no symptoms is dangerous.

There are also the uncounted thousands of drug users who inject themselves using contaminated syringes, not just in the American ghettoes, but even in northeast India near the Burmese border, where there is a huge refugee crisis and few sterile syringes.[3] And what about all the children who suffer in this pandemic? Hundreds of thousands have been effectively orphaned when their single-mother parents died from AIDS contracted from partners who did not stick around to help raise their children. AIDS is also one of the infections that can be passed to a foetus *in utero* through the placenta during pregnancy, or at the time of birth or in breast milk. The last route can be avoided by using formula milk for the infant, but many Third World mothers are too poor to buy it, or have no source of clean water with which to prepare it. Under-fives figure largely in the group with the highest fatality. Overall, the HIV pandemic is estimated at the time of writing to have caused the deaths of 32 million people and to be infecting 40 million others, including 2.5 million children. The UN Population Division predicts deaths from HIV to reach 300 million in the next half-century.[4]

Bejel is an infectious disease similar to syphilis, but transmitted by mouth-to-mouth contact or sharing eating and drinking utensils, especially between children in poor countries, not necessarily by sexual activity. It is categorised as a nonvenereal spirochetal infection, caused by the spirochete *triponema pallidum endemicum* and is successfully treatable with penicillin. Bejel occurs mainly in hot, dry regions of the eastern Mediterranean basin and West Africa. It begins as a painless patch on the mucous membrane of the mouth or at the angles of the lips, which touch a shared cup. These may disappear and be followed by lesions on the trunk, legs and arms, in turn followed by gummatous lesions, similar to syphilitic lesions in the nose and soft palate.

First identified by German physician Theodor Bilharz (1825–1862), **Bilharzia** is also known as schistosomiasis and colloquially as snail fever. It is caused by parasitic *schistosoma* flatworms invading the human urinary tract or intestines and producing abdominal pain, diarrhoea, bloody stools and blood in the urine. In time it can also cause liver damage, kidney failure, infertility and bladder cancer. The reservoir is in infected freshwater snails living in slow-moving water courses or canals. Children are particularly at risk if they play in this water. Other high-risk groups include farmers, fishermen, and people using the affected water for drinking or washing. Diagnosis is by identifying eggs of the parasite in a sick person's urine or stool, or by detecting antibodies in a blood sample. In areas where bilharzia is common, WHO recommends an annual prophylactic dose by mouth of the drug praziquantel, which is also used to treat those already infected.

Bilharzia affects about 252 million people of the 700 million living in the danger areas of Africa, Asia and South America, with as many as 200,000 dying from the disease each year. Many victims experience nothing more than 'swimmer's itch' at first or a slight rash lasting for several days. Other symptoms presenting two to ten weeks later include fever and chills, general aches and pains, coughing, diarrhoea and enlarged glands. If eggs of the worms migrate to the brain or spinal cord, seizures, paralysis and other unpleasant neurological symptoms can be added.

Acute schistosomiasis, called *katayama* fever, causes fever, urticaria, rashes, liver and spleen enlargement and bronchospasm. Women may suffer genital lesions making them prone to a high risk of HIV transmission. Infected people release *schistosoma* eggs into water via their fecal material or urine. Larvae from these eggs infect freshwater snails and reproduce there, leaving the snail to live briefly in the water, where it must find a mammalian host within forty-eight hours, or die. Bilharzia has been around a long time; in 2014 remains of an Egyptian child who died 6,200 years ago showed evidence of it. It was so widespread there that, until the twentieth century, blood in the urine of Egyptian boys was viewed as male menstruation and perfectly normal.

From its origin in Africa, the **chikungunya** arbovirus, a member of the genus *alphavirus* of the family *togaviridae*, has come a long way in the bodies of travellers who acquired it by the bite of female *aedes aegypti* and *aedes albopictus* mosquitoes, themselves infected when taking a blood meal from an infected human in numerous countries of Africa, Asia and islands in the Indian and Pacific Oceans. In Europe, so far the risk only exists in France and Italy. In 2013 the virus was found for the first time on islands in the Caribbean and is now endemic in Florida and Brazil, the latter counting almost 1 million cases now.

If, on arrival in their own country, infected travellers allow themselves to be bitten by a local mosquito, chikungunya will rapidly become an epidemic there, as it did when first detected in the Western hemisphere on the Caribbean island of St Marten in October 2013. Within the year, it had covered the hemisphere. There is no vaccine to prevent or medicine to treat chikungunya virus infection, but travellers can protect themselves and other people by preventing mosquito bites. They are advised to use insect repellent, wear long sleeves and trousers, not to wear sandals without socks, and to stay in accommodation with air conditioning or with window and door screens and nets over the beds.

The most common symptoms of infection that develop between three and seven days from the mosquito bites are fever and joint pain, which may be accompanied by headache, muscle pain, swollen joints or a rash, severe and disabling and usually lasting a week. In some cases the symptoms endure for months. The outcome is not usually fatal, except for infants, the elderly and those with pre-existing conditions like high blood pressure, diabetes or heart disease. There is no specific treatment, but good medical advice is to rest, drink a lot of fluids and use paracetamol to smother the pain.

The common names for **dengue fever** include 'the vomiting fever'; the most menacing is 'breakbone fever'. In the West Indies, African slaves who were infected had such pain in their bones and joints that they were said to walk like an effete dandy; hence another common name, 'dandy fever'. Symptoms include severe headaches, muscle, joint and bone pain, skin rashes and haemorhagic shows like bleeding from gums and body orifices. Under whatever name, dengue is said to be caused by one of five positive-stranded RNA viruses of the *flaviviridae* family, although, alarmingly, some researchers say there are forty-seven of them. Vectored by infected female *aedes aegypti* mosquitoes, these pathogens are estimated to cause 390 million infections each year in tropical countries lying in southern Asia and Central and South America during the rainy season. Incubation after the mosquito bite may be anything from three to fourteen days, after which the fever lasts between three days and a week, unless it becomes severe, when it can be lethal.

The victims are not contagious. Although confusingly many are asymptomatic, dengue can cause severe haemorrhagic fever and shock syndrome. While many victims suffer simultaneous infection by *zikavirus* and *chikungunya*, patients with simple dengue fever usually recover in ten to fifteen days. The traditional cure for dengue fever was juice made from the crushed leaves of the papaya fruit. Only one vaccine for dengue has so far been synthesised in laboratories, and is legally used in Singapore, Thailand, Indonesia, seven South American countries and the Philippines. A problem here is that it treats only one of the four types of dengue and, if a cured patient is subsequently infected with one of the other types, the antibodies from the first infection may actually enhance the virulence of the new form of the virus, producing haemorrhagic fever, with symptoms persisting for several months. Similarly, dengue-infected women who have babies pass on their specific immunity to the infants, who then risk haemorrhagic fever if infected with one of the other types. The French pharmaceutical giant Sanofi has produced a four-serotype vaccine called Denvaxia, used in several countries for patients in the 9 to 45 years age-bracket. For whatever reasons, the American Food and Drugs Administration only approves it for 9 to 16-year-olds on US territory.

Because most victims of tropical diseases are not able to express themselves in European languages, it is rare to have an account from a sufferer of dengue fever. In 1942 war reporter Martha Gellhorn was exploring in the Dutch colony of Surinam on the north coast of South America. As an adventure, she hired a dugout canoe and a crew of paddlers to take her upstream through dense jungle on the Saramacca River into uncharted territory, where natives in river bank villages demonstrated their animosity with showers of missiles. It being unwise to step ashore, she and the crew ate, performed all their bodily functions and slept in the dugout canoe. With no protection from the swarms of mosquitoes that invaded the boat each night, she was severely bitten by female *aedes* mosquitoes and went down with dengue. On the fifth day of what had turned into a nightmare expedition, she was shivering in high fever and unable to move normally, such was the pain in her joints. Thrashing about in the boat, semi-conscious, she fractured a wrist. Seeing that her ankles were grossly swollen, she feared that she had elephantiasis. The boat turned around, it was paddled downstream with the current, stopping at the first township that had a Dutch doctor, who diagnosed dengue fever and treated her.[5]

Although a tall, leggy blonde who dressed very expensively when not wearing uniform to be protected by the rules of war, Gellhorn was no pampered denizen of the fashionable cocktail bars, but shared the hardships of her male colleagues in the field uncomplainingly, expecting no special treatment. She had already covered several wars and was used to freezing conditions during winter in the mountains while covering the Spanish civil war and being shelled and sniped at while sheltering for days and nights on end in flooded trenches. She was, in a word, tough. Yet dengue reduced her to a shivering, helpless creature.

Ebola fever is caused by another filovirus and is zoonotic, the reservoir being in African fruit bats and chimpanzees and forest antelopes, hunted for food. Primary infection takes place in humans who eat poorly cooked bushmeat, but contact with them can pass the infection person-to-person. Ebola fever was first identified during 1976 in Zaire (now Democratic Republic of Congo) near the Ebola river. Yet the second confirmed outbreak occurred on the other side of Africa, 1,000 miles away in the

Sudan. The good news is that US Food and Drug Administration has approved a vaccine designated VSV-ZEBOV and commercialised as Ervebo; but the bad news is that this is effective only against the Zaire ebolavirus and there are three other major variants of virulent Ebola, for which it is ineffective: *Sudan ebolavirus; Taï Forest (or Côte d'Ivoire) ebolavirus* and *Bundibugyo ebolavirus*. Two other variants designated *reston ebolavirus* and *bombali ebolavirus* also exist out there in fruit bat and other zoonotic reservoirs, but do not so far affect humans.

People are infected through contact with blood, body fluids like urine, faeces, sweat, breast milk and semen that penetrate victims' broken skin or enter their bodies through the mucous membrane of the eyes, nose or mouth, the digestive tract and sexual organs. Ebola also infects people handling the corpses of those who died, or relatives who 'inherit' the deceased's clothing or blankets impregnated with the virus in areas of extreme poverty. Symptoms starting with fever, aches and pains, then progressing to diarrhoea, vomiting and uncontrollable bleeding lead to death in anywhere between two and twenty-one days. Like Covid-19, ebolavirus can survive on hard surfaces for days unless they are intensively sterilised by powerful hospital-grade disinfectants

Recovery from Ebola requires a good immune reaction as well as specialist nursing care. Survivors show signs of antibodies several years after being ill. One especially chilling characteristic is that, even in sufferers who have been treated and are apparently clear, the virus can 'hide' in the testes, inside the eyes, in the placenta and within the central nervous system in the cerebrospinal fluid. So unprotected sex with a person who has apparently recovered is highly inadvisable. Obviously, health care workers need to exercise extreme caution when dealing with victims of Ebola, and must use head-to-toe disposable protective clothing and masks, burnt after use. The 2014–16 outbreak in Guinea turned into an epidemic in other West African states claiming more than 11,000 lives. This was partly due to local, untrained nursing personnel in a remote area of southeast Guinea re-using their entire stock of a half-dozen hypodermic needles to treat 300 patients. Eleven outbreaks occurred in Democratic Republic of Congo where the inadequate health infrastructure has to cope with other endemic infectious tropical diseases and malnutrition caused by armed conflict.

In February 2021 the government of Guinea announced that it had a new outbreak on its hands, apparently due to the custom of community funerals, when neighbours and friends help to wash the body of the deceased. In this case, after the death of a nurse working in a health centre near Nzérékoré on 28 February seven people attending the burial contracted Ebola. That is within walking distance of the porous frontiers with Liberia and Ivory Coast. The WHO representative in Guinea reported that an Ebola vaccine was trialled in the country for four months in 2015 and other new drugs are available that can increase the survival chances of those infected. As a result, eleven outbreaks have been suppressed before reaching epidemic level in the Democratic Republic of Congo.

Respected freelance reporter Umaru Fofana in Sierra Leone says there is far more fear of Ebola in that country than of Covid-19. Although the vaccine alliance Gavi has access to a global stockpile of 500,000 doses, should that prove insufficient, there could be a problem because the vaccine manufacturers are concentrating on Covid-19 drugs.

The **hantaviridae group of viruses** was first noted during the Korean war (1950–53) when 3,000 fit and well-fed United Nations troops fell ill with symptoms that included extreme fatigue, fever, muscle pain, headaches, dizziness, nausea, vomiting, diarrhoea and severe respiratory symptoms. The particular virus in question was identified only more than two decades later in 1978 when the etiologic agent of this Korean haemorrhagic fever – sometimes presenting as a pulmonary infection or kidney disease – was identified in field rodents of the species *apodemus agrarius* in the valley of the Hantaan River, a tributary of the Injin in the north of South Korea.

Some of the returning soldiers carried this virus back with them when rotated home, and the hantavirus which causes severe pulmonary distress in humans and bleeding in the kidneys is now endemic in rodents in the Four Corners area of southwestern USA. The virus is in the bodily fluids and excrement of infected rodents. The vector in this case is not a flea but instinctive human tidiness: when sweeping up rodent droppings, some of the contaminated dust is inhaled by the sweeper, unless he/she is wearing a mask. That's all it takes. One case that horrified the well-known biologist Christopher Wills was a student of his who was carrying out a survey of birdlife in the Sierra Nevada mountains of California. Apparently not alarmed that it was infested with fieldmice, she made her temporary base in a remote cabin that had been empty for several months. Inhaling dust from their droppings killed her.[6]

Hantavirus pulmonary syndrome occurs in rural areas of the United States during spring and summer months, also in South America and Canada – a whole range of climatic conditions. An outbreak in the Four Corners region during November 1993 was investigated at the US Center for Disease Control using tissue taken from a deer mouse trapped near the home of a victim. About one in five deer mice are infected, but rarely infect humans because the virus is killed by sunlight and there are no known cases of person-to-person transfer. Alternatively, a 10 per cent solution of bleach completely destroys this virus. The disease usually clears up after a few days, causing no residual complications.

Lassa fever is a viral haemorrhagic fever, for which no vaccine exists, named after the town of Lassa in Borno State, Nigeria. The population of the town is most unhappy about this because, although this disease is relatively common in other West African countries like Liberia, Sierra Leone, Guinea, Ghana and also some regions of Nigeria, the first case recorded in the town itself in 1969 was not a local person, but a retired nurse working for the American missionary organisation Church of the Brethren named Ms. Laura Wine. Soon after her return from leave in the US to her post as head of obstetrics at the Mission Hospital in Lassa, she came down with a fever and was taken to the general hospital there, where she was treated for malaria. This had no effect, so the Lassa hospital contacted what is now Bingham University Teaching Hospital, a bigger and better equipped health centre in the town of Jos, ten hours' drive away. They sent a light aircraft to transfer her there more quickly, so she could have better medical attention than was available in Lassa.

Despite this, her symptoms worsened and Ms Wine died. Shortly afterwards the doctor and nurse who had been treating her also died, proving that the fever was highly contagious. Samples sent to the US CDC indicated that the virus was previously unknown there, but belonged to the group known as arenaviruses from the Latin *arena* meaning sand because they have a sandy appearance under the microscope. Other viruses in the group have been known since 1933 and are found in South America and Africa. Meanwhile, another nurse died in Lassa, probably infected by contact with Ms Wine.

The hunt was on. Backtracking her return route to Nigeria, doctors discovered that she had returned to Lassa by travelling through another West African country, which was probably Sierra Leone. It seems she picked up the virus there, where it is zoonotic, the reservoir being in rats of the species *mastomys natalensis*, which frequent villages and towns and whose urine and faeces contain the virus, which may be deposited on dishes and cups in households with poor hygiene, or even in the food and water supplies. Humans coming into contact with the virus develop the fever and themselves transmit it to other humans through their blood, urine, faeces and other body secretions. A common symptom is deafness, occurring in one in three infected people, although many of the natives infected show no symptoms, presumably because the rats have been around for many generations, enabling the local inhabitants to acquire a level of immunity. The antiviral drug *ribavirin* can cure Lassa fever, if given early enough. Infected tourists who fail to be treated, are likely to die.

Leishmaniasis is a disease that afflicted crusaders in the Holy Land eight centuries ago, and is still a current threat in tropical and subtropical countries and in Southern Europe. The only continent where it is not found is Australia, which has rigorous border controls to prevent its installation. It is also not a threat in Antarctica, for reasons that will become obvious. The vector is the female phlebotomine sand fly, from which one bite may suffice to infect the careless tourist who sleeps rough, wanders about after dusk, wears sandals or fails to tuck shirt into trousers or cover the legs with trousers tucked into socks. Insect-proof nets, and clothing pre-treated with pyrethroid insecticide should be purchased before visiting territories where these sand flies are found. The parasite they inject when biting a human for a blood meal is one or other of the Leishmania pathogens. There are quite a few variations.

Because a sand fly is so small – one quarter the size of a mosquito – this dangerous insect is often not even seen by its victims. So, insect repellent containing DEET chemicals should be used prophylactically under the cuffs of shirt sleeves and on the ankles. The same advice as for mosquitoes is to stay in air-conditioned or screened accommodation, spray your room with insecticide and use a similarly treated bed net, tucked well in under the mattress. In the Western hemisphere, the danger zone includes Mexico, Central and South America, but not yet Chile or Uruguay, for whatever reason. Some cases have been found in Texas and Oklahoma, the Leishmania parasites that infect local sand flies having travelled back with tourists returning from Latin America. Flies can also acquire the parasites from infected rodents or domestic pets.

174

The most common form of the disease caused by some of the twenty or more species of the parasite is cutaneous leishmaniasis, presenting as skin sores on a million or more people per annum. These usually heal without treatment, sometimes after months or longer, but can leave ugly scars. Another risk is for cutaneous leishmaniasis to go mucocutaneous, spreading to the mucous membrane of the nose, mouth or throat – sometimes long after the skin sores have healed – so early treatment is advised. Even worse is visceral leishmaniasis, also called *kala*-azar, which can attack internal organs: spleen, liver and even bone marrow. Untreated, it can be fatal.

A whole group of tiny, ultra-thin pathogens are known as filoviruses, meaning thread-like viruses. The first detected, **Marburg virus** was named for the West German town where technicians involved in the production of poliomyelitis vaccine at the Behringwerke laboratory in 1967 fell ill after handling without adequate precautions body tissues taken from infected African green monkeys. Also infected were employees of the Paul Ehrlich Institute in Frankfurt doing similar research with the same consignment of animals. The first technicians infected were treated in their homes for up to ten days, suffering symptoms of extreme malaise, myalgia, crippling headaches, with temperatures as high as 39°C (102.2F). Although the clinical symptoms were not very alarming during the first three or four days, additional symptoms subsequently appeared, including nausea, vomiting, and diarrhoea so severe that health care professionals treating them suspected dysentery or typhoid fever. When these were ruled out after testing in hospital, the patients' temperatures fell to 38°C, and they developed petechiae and more severe signs of internal hemorrhaging with bleeding from all bodily orifices and even from the minute skin punctures made by hypodermic needles.

Marburg virus in humans can produce, in addition to the symptoms mentioned above, abdominal pain, inflammation of the pancreas, liver failure, massive internal bleeding and multiple organ dysfunction. Endemic in primates in Democratic Republic of Congo, Angola, Gabon, Kenya and other zones of Africa, the virus's historic vector for infecting humans was by bats in sub-Saharan Africa infecting monkeys that were then killed and eaten as inadequately cooked bush meat with 80 per cent fatalities among the consumers. Death usually occurs eight or nine days after infection, preceded by severe blood loss and shock. There is no known cure, but testing of samples in disease control centres with ultra-screened Biosafety Level 4 laboratories can identify MARV infection.

The zoonotic reservoir of this pathogen is in colonies of the African fruit bat *rousettus aegyptiacus* which roost in caves and disused mines, each colony having as many as 100,000 bats that emerge each night to go foraging, feeding on fruit in close contact with monkeys who live in the treetops, possibly also biting them to obtain blood. Person-to-person transmission happens subsequently when previously unaffected people have contact with the blood or other body fluids of infected animals or humans, or their clothing or bedding. Notable outbreaks include Belgrade in 1967, Angola in 2005, Congo in 1998–2008, Uganda in 2012 and Kenya in 1980–87.

The three European occurrences in 1967 at Marburg, Frankfurt and Belgrade had a common source in a single consignment of monkeys imported from Uganda, destination Frankfurt. In an indirect effect of the Six-Day War in June 1967, the monkeys were diverted to London airport and kept in an animal house there for two days before being forwarded to Frankfurt airport, with some onforwarded to Belgrade. Two monkeys escaped from the animal house in London airport and were recovered after several days of liberty, but did not infect any person or animal in their wanderings. The monkeys arriving at the laboratories in Frankfurt and Marburg appeared healthy and were killed immediately to extract kidney tissues. Those sent to Belgrade's Institute Torlak were kept alive there for six weeks before being killed and their organs harvested.

Later, it was found that when Ugandan monkey trappers caught obviously sick animals that could not be sold to European laboratories, they isolated them on an island in Lake Victoria, to die or survive without infecting other animals. However, when lacking enough monkeys to complete a shipment, they returned to the island and trapped some *healthy-looking* animals to include in the shipment. At the time of the Marburg and Frankfurt cases, however, the African origin of the pathogen could not be proven because it *could* have been picked up when the monkeys were in the London airport animal house or when the two monkeys escaped.

Eight years later, an Australian backpacker who had been hitchhiking in Zimbabwe with a woman companion fell ill in Johannesburg, South Africa, and died a few days after admission to hospital. His companion and a nurse developed milder symptoms and recovered. Samples taken from them proved to contain a strain of Marburg similar to that of the 1967 monkeys. Further cases of the disease were all traceable to the couple's recent visit to East Africa – a good place not to go!

Related to SARS (q.v.), the virus causing **Middle East respiratory syndrome** (MERS) thrives in Saudi Arabia and other countries of the region, its vector being bats that have taken blood meals from camels. Many tourists are persuaded to take camel rides for fun, unaware that the animals cough and dribble, propelling droplets all around and causing MERS in the unwary.

The virus causing the **severe acute respiratory syndrome** (SARS) labelled as Cov-1, emerged from Guangdong province in China during November 2002 and travelled by droplet infection in two years to thirty other countries killing nearly 10 per cent of its victims, mainly in Asia.

Pigs are often kept penned up in close contact with each other under intensive factory conditions, with thousands under one roof. They are particularly susceptible to droplet-spread virus infections which they, in turn, can pass on to humans as **swine fever**. In tropical countries, pigs are often confined at night underneath the elevated houses of their owners, who sleep on the woven palm leaf floor. A layer of woven palm leaves is no barrier to the virus, which penetrates it easily, to be inhaled by the people above.

Pigs and humans are genetically similar, enabling viruses to jump between the two animal species. Is that why so many peoples – Jews, Muslims and Hindus among them – have a long-standing ban on keeping pigs and eating pork? Son Hong Lei of China's Centre for Control and Prevention of Disease and Liu Jin Haa of the Chinese Agricultural University presented a report in June 2020 on the risk of swine fever affecting humans.[7] They had traced 179 viruses with this potential, of which variant G4 EA H1N1 combines three lines of descent, making it very potent.

Leading Thai virologist Dr Yong Poovorawan agrees with the two Chinese researchers that if this mutated virus jumps from pigs to people, they would be unlikely to have any immunity, so that it could provoke a new pandemic. In the US Dr Anthony Fauci, director of the National Institute of Allergy and Infectious Diseases told the Senate that the new virus is being closely monitored because it shares similar properties with the H1N1 virus of 2009 and the pandemic of Spanish 'flu in 1918–20. A report on the digital news portal *Asia One* argues that people working in the pork industry should be closely monitored because tests have shown that the new virus has established itself and reproduced in cells of the human respiratory tract. Dr Amesh Adalja of Johns Hopkins Centre for Health Security commented, 'This is one of the 'flu viruses we'll have to keep close track of.'

In a parallel scare, the Danish Prime Minister Mette Frederiksen, in consultation with WHO and the European Centre for Disease Prevention and Control, announced in November 2020 that all 17 million mink being bred for their fur in Danish factory farms were to be killed, and presumably incinerated because some of the animals had caught Covid-19 from their human handlers. The minks' metabolism had produced a mutation in the coronavirus that, if it were to jump back to humans, would probably not respond to the Covid-19 vaccine being made at the time of writing this chapter. British truckers attempting to return from Denmark were refused entry to the UK. Across the world every country with mink farms was instructed by WHO to kill and incinerate every single animal.

The vector for the *trypanosoma brucei* protozoan parasites that cause the disease commonly called **sleeping sickness** and properly called tripanosomiasis is the tsetse fly (*glossina morsitans*), which lives in twenty-five countries of sub-Saharan Africa. It acquires the parasites when biting infected humans or animals like cattle. The parasite can also be transmitted from mother to child during pregnancy if the trypanosome crosses the placental barrier and infects the foetus. Identified by French naval surgeon Marie-Théophile Griffon du Bellay while serving in Gabon during the late 1860s, the life cycle and vector were not known for certain until half a century later. The disease went epidemic in 1896–1906, 1920 and again in the late 1990s. Currently, the vast majority of cases are in the Democratic Republic of Congo. Treatment during the first stage of human infection by pentamidine in West Africa and suramin in East Africa has few side effects and is easy to administer.

Initial symptoms include fever, severe headaches, irritability, extreme fatigue, swollen lymph nodes, rashes and pain in muscles and joints. Untreated, the disease is fatal after it invades the central nervous system by crossing the blood-brain barrier, causing confusion, tremors and poor coordination, ataxia, speech problems, numbness and loss of muscle tone, personality changes and other neurological problems leading to coma and death. In the East African form, *trypanosoma brucei rhodesiense* kills within months; the West African *trypanosoma brucei gambiense* may take years. Sleeping sickness existed in isolated pockets in Africa for thousands of years. What caused the spread of tripanosomiasis was the arrival in Central and West Africa of Arab slave traders from the east of the continent, who brought the parasites with them.

Almost nobody had ever heard of **West Nile Fever** until it was first diagnosed in one woman living in the West Nile district of Uganda in 1937, since when many cases in humans have been reported in various countries. The fever itself remained a bit of a mystery until the virus was identified in 1953, vectored by mosquitoes on crows and pigeons in the Nile delta, which it did not seem to harm. In 1997 a more virulent strain of the virus was found to be causing encephalitis and paralysis in different avian species in Israel. From there, this pathogen – a single-stranded RNA virus of the flaviviridae group, which includes Zika virus, dengue virus and yellow fever virus – produced an explosive outbreak in New York in 1999, which spread throughout the United States 1999–2010, becoming the most common arboviral infection in North America. Its spread north to Canada and south to Latin America illustrates just how fast a vector-borne pathogen can spread when carried by international travellers outside its historic habitat. Avian travellers with feathers also carried it along their annual migratory routes to Greece, Romania, Russia, Western Asia and Australia.

Some 20 per cent of human sufferers develop some of these symptoms: fever of 38.3C (101F), headaches (because the virus can cause inflammation of brain tissue and interfere with the functioning of the central nervous system), inflamed hair follicles, irritation of the eyes, joint and muscle pain, vomiting, diarrhoea, skin rashes like measles and swollen lymph nodes. They present between two to six days after the bite of a mosquito that has taken blood from an infected bird, but the incubation period can be as long as twenty-one days. Severe cases may also suffer torticollis (stiff neck), dangerous drowsiness that makes driving unwise, a sense of disorientation, tremors, convulsions, paralysis, coma and, rarely, encephalitis or meningitis. Recovery may leave the patients suffering post-viral fatigue and weakness lasting for months, as well as speech and memory problems. As much as 15 per cent of severe cases *can* prove fatal. Alarmingly, in the state of Texas what seems to be a modified strain of WNF virus is, like the AIDS virus, able to block a cell's ability to summon help from the body's immune system.

Yaws is a disease that has been around a long time, fossil evidence suggesting it was present in ancestors of humans living 1.6 million years ago. It is currently an endemic infection in fifteen or more tropical countries under many different local names, and is particularly prevalent in Ghana, New Guinea and the Solomon Islands. Yaws affects the skin, the bones and the joints. The spirochete bacterium *triponema pallidum pertenue* invades the body through small lesions like the scratches from walking through undergrowth or long grass. Incubation can be as fast as nine days or as slow as ninety days, but is usually around three weeks. Although it is not transmitted sexually, some of the symptoms resemble those of endemic syphilis or *bejel* – as which it is sometimes misdiagnosed – and *pinta* in Central and South America, which is not very contagious. First symptom is a hard, round swelling under the skin one inch or larger in diameter.

The Spanish name *frambesia* is derived from *frambuesa* meaning raspberry because when a papule under the armpit or in other areas of moist skin bursts, it releases a highly infectious exudate, leaving the surface resembling the appearance of a raspberry. Nearby lymph nodes may be swollen and tender to the touch. Secondary yaws develops more slowly, sometimes even months after infection, and is noted for pain in the long bones and fingers, which can be distorted and mis-shapen in 10 per cent of cases. Painful lesions may also develop on the palms of the hands and the soles of the feet, called crab yaws. Sooner or later, an assortment of unsightly, painful and disfiguring lesions and facial ulcers may appear, particularly around the nose and on the limbs. Developing into large, protruding whitish crusted sores with necrotic flesh that are particularly noticeable on black skin, they are like a warning to keep clear.

Global attempts to eradicate yaws in the 1950s and in 2012 having failed, it continues to target children under 15 for the most part. Left untreated, it is a disfiguring and debilitating disease, but it can be cured with a single dose of the cheap antibiotic azithromycin, taken orally, although the bacterium seems to be acquiring antibiotic resistance. Alternatively, a single intramuscular injection of benzathine penicillin with some risk of anaphylactic shock, may do the trick. It is currently believed that the reservoir of this unpleasant condition is in humans, with transmission by person-to-person contact, impossible to avoid in areas where a whole family may live in a one-room dwelling. So rats, mice and mosquitoes are not to blame. Rather, poverty, poor living conditions and bad personal hygiene are what keep yaws thriving. Radically improving hygiene and sanitation can clear a whole community. Unfortunately, this happens rarely in tropical Third World countries.

In Europe, **yellow fever** was observed in Lisbon in 1723 and also later in Spain, having presumably been brought back from the Latin-American territories claimed by the two monarchies. It also visited the port of Southampton and Swansea in Wales in 1777. The last cases in Europe seem to have been in 1908 at the port of St Nazaire in Brittany, with seven fatalities. In tropical Central and South America, yellow fever has been known as a killer for centuries, having fatally afflicted pirates of the Caribbean, *conquistadores* and missionary priests during and after the Spanish conquests. It owes the name to the jaundice produced before the death of the victim, although some say it is from the yellow jack or flag displayed by ships in quarantine, signalling infection on board. The author first came across this disease when writing a history of the French Foreign Legion.

President Abraham Lincoln (elected 1861, assassinated 1865) was the intended victim of a plot by Confederate sympathiser Dr Luke Blackburn to infect him with yellow fever in the summer of 1864. Not knowing the true vector of the virus, Blackburn took clothing of deceased victims that was stained with their vomited blood and packed them together in a trunk with new clothes, thinking that they would make the new ones infectious. Based in Toronto, Ontario, he commissioned another man to take the clothes across the US border into Union territory and have the trunk delivered to the White House in the hope that Lincoln would wear the new clothes in it. More of the supposedly contaminated clothes were to be auctioned in Union territory, to infect as many people as possible. The whole plan unravelled because Blackburn refused to pay his agent when they next met in Toronto, so angering the man that he walked into the office of the US consul and exposed the whole plot in exchange for a guarantee of immunity and a cash payment. Where this might have led, we do not know because two days later President Lincoln was assassinated by actor John Wilkes Booth while watching a performance of *Our American Cousin* at Ford's Theatre in Washington.

However, yellow fever persists in Africa and South America, both in remote areas and in the towns. In the country, it seems that monkeys were the first choice for the *aedes aegypti mosquitoes in Africa* and the species *haemagogus* and *sabethes* in South America and the Caribbean. Strangely, the urban form is the more serious. Eradication programmes concentrate on eliminating stagnant water or treating the surface of it with anti-mosquito sprays. Visitors to yellow fever countries are usually required to have a prophylactic injection before travel with a cheap and effective vaccine, of which one dose suffices to give lifelong immunity.

Zika fever comes from the Ziika forest in Uganda, where this virus was first identified in a monkey in 1947 and detected in a mosquito several months later. One of Zika's nastiest symptoms is that unprotected contact between a woman who is pregnant or intending to become so and an infected sexual partner can cause microcephaly in the foetus and other irreversible brain malformations and birth defects. Women can also pass zikavirus to their sexual partners. In April 2016 the Institut Pasteur in Paris recorded 196 cases in metropolitan France including seven pregnant women.

Zika is an arbovirus, spread by the bite of arthropods like ticks and the female *aedes aegypti* mosquito. *Aedes albopictus*, a species increasingly found in Europe, is commonly known as the Asiatic tiger mosquito, another vector. Zika's natural habitat lies in a spread of equatorial countries of Africa and Asia. The US Center for Disease Control issued travel advice to women of childbearing age, not to travel to these countries because of the risks, but after 2007 the virus ZIKV was carried by travellers to the Americas and passed by them to local mosquitoes, who then passed it back to other humans. In 2015–16 there were extensive outbreaks in North America, particularly in Florida and Texas, but since 2019 the risk there has considerably reduced, although Zika is alive and well in Central and South America and across the Pacific islands, thus girdling the planet. Eight out of ten victims experience no, or only mild, symptoms, but even so travellers should ensure they do not get bitten by local mosquitoes for several weeks after returning home, just in case. Incubation lasts between three and twelve days, after which severe symptoms *may* be due to neurological damage leading as far as paralysis of the respiratory muscles. There is no vaccine or treatment for Zika, although pain-killers and anti-inflammatory medication can relieve some symptoms. Exposure to mosquitoes is often due to tourists wearing inappropriately scanty clothing in the daytime or sleeping with open and unscreened windows at night and failing to use mosquito nets over their beds.

What can be done to contain Zika? The answer is a military one: to poison all the mosquitoes' still-water egg-laying sites by spraying on them oily toxic products which float on the surface. Aerial spraying by fixed-wing aircraft and helicopters is the most effective method. No mosquitoes = no Zika. Of course, in impoverished Third World countries there may be no funds for this, but international agencies are in many cases stepping into the breach for the common good.

Acknowledgements

As a historian with no formal medical training, I could not have written this book without help. My thanks go to David I. Ben-Tovim, Professor of Psychiatry and Clinical Epidemiology at Flinders University, Adelaide, South Australia, for taking the time to read through the draft text and make comments that led me to numerous paths of enquiry that I should never have found. Not all of them could be included in the final text, so any errors and omissions are mine alone.

The photograph of Justinian I was taken by Petar Milošević (CC BY-SA, Wikipedia), for whose permission to publish I am most grateful. The other illustrations are from the author's collection. For digging up much grist to the author's mill, I thank my wife Atarah and our friend Jennifer Weller. At Pen and Sword Publications, I also acknowledge the encouragement and professional skills of Series Editor Dr Danna R. Messer, Commissioning Editor Claire Hopkins and Production Editor Laura Hirst.

Further Reading

K. Alibek and S. Handelman, *Biohazard*, New York: Dell Publishing 2000

C. Arnold, *Pandemic 1918*, New York: Macmillan 2018

R. Boulton, *An Essay on the Plague*, Farmington Hills: Gale ECCO Print Editions 2010

N. Cummins, M. Kelly and C. Ó Gráda, 'Living Standards and Plague in London 1560–1665', *English Historical Review* 69 (1), pp. 3 – 34, downloadable from http://prints.lse.ac.uk/65092

The Diary of John Evelyn, ed. W. Bray, Delhi, Lector House, no date

The Diary of Samuel Pepys (all entries) downloadable from www.pepysdiary.com/diary/

J. Kelly, *The Great Mortality: An Intimate History of the Black Death*, London: Harper Perennial 2013

W.H. Mc Neill, *Plagues and Peoples*, New York: Anchor Books 1998

D.Pua, D. Dybbro and A. Rogers, *Unit 731: The Forgotten Asian Auschwitz*, second edition, privately printed

C. Scott and C. Duncan, *Return of the Black Death*, Chichester: Wiley and Sons 2004

P. Slack, *The Impact of Plague in Tudor and Stuart England*, Oxford: Clarendon Press 1991

C. Wills, *Plagues*, London: HarperCollins 1916

E.A. Wrigley and R.S. Schofield, *The Population History of England 1541–1871*, London: Hodder & Stoughton 1981

P. Ziegler, *The Black Death* London, Penguin 1982

H. Zinsser, *Rats, Lice and History*, London: Penguin 2000

Notes and Sources

Chapter 1

1. W.H. McNeill, *Plagues and Peoples*, New York: Anchor Books 1998, p. 36
2. Ibid, p. 37.
3. Philipp Wolfgang Stockhammer et al (eds), *The Stone Age Plague: 1,000 years of Persistence in Eurasia*, 2016, downloaded by courtesy of Academia website. Likewise *The Long and Complicated Relationship between Humans and Yersinia Pestis* – a senior honours thesis by Sterling Wright at the University of Texas at Austin 2016.
4. See Rasmussen et al, *Early Divergent Strains of Yersinia Pestis in Eurasia 5,000 Years Ago*, downloadable from http://dx.doi.org/10.1016/j.cell.2015.10.009.
5. C. Wills, *Plagues: Their Origin, History and Future*, London: Harper Collins 1996, pp. 11, 14.
6. Ibid, p. 92.
7. Ibid, pp. 95-7.
8. Report in *The Lancet*, vol. 383 of 2014.
9. See Wright, *The Long and Complicated Relationship between Humans and Yersinia Pestis* for more technical information.
10. Ibid.
11. Book of Numbers 25.
12. Wills, *Plagues*, pp. 69,70.

Chapter 2

1. *Plague Manuel: Epidemiology, Distribution, Surveillance and Control* Geneva, WHO 1999, pp. 23-4.
2. A copy of this very first peace treaty is displayed at the headquarters of UNO in New York.

3. The term exodus is Greek for departure. In Hebrew, this book is called *Shemot* – the names.
4. See archive.archaelogy.org/online/news/karameikos.html.
5. So called from the family name of Emperor Marcus Aurelius Antoninus.
6. It is sometimes called the plague of Galen.
7. McNeill, *Plagues and Peoples*, p. 126.
8. Ibid, p. 128.
9. K. Chimin Wong and Wu Lien-Te *History of Chinese Medicine, Being a Chronicle of Medical Happenings in China from Ancient Times to the Present Period*, Shanghai 1936, p. 28, quoted in McNeill, *Plagues and Peoples*, p. 146.
10. Cyprian's works may be found in J-P Migne's *Patrologia Latina* Vols 3 & 4, Paris 1844.
11. http://sourcebooks.fordham.edu/source/542procopius-plague.asp (abridged).
12. S. Scott and C.J. Duncan, *Return of the Black Death*, Chichester: J. Wiley & Sons 2004, p. 237.
13. Ch'en Kao-Yung *Chung Kao Li Tai Tien Tsai Jen Huo Piao* published in two volumes at Shanghai 1940.
14. Quoted in McNeill, *Plagues and Peoples*, pp. 297-301.
15. Article by Arthur Boylston in the *Journal of the Royal Society of Medicine*, July 2012.
16. Article by Timothy P. Newfield in the *Journal of Interdisciplinary History* 46 (Summer 2015), pp. 1-38.
17. H. Zinsser, *Rats, Lice and History*, London: Penguin 2000, pp. 150-5.

Chapter 3

1. McNeill, *Plagues and Peoples*, p. 163.
2. Article by M. Moore in *Daily Telegraph* 1 November 2010.
3. J. Kelly, *The Great Mortality*, London: Harper Perennial 2013, pp. 3-5.
4. Ibid, p. 6.
5. J.P. Byrne, *Encyclopedia of the Black Death*, Santa Barbara: ABC-CLIO 2012, p. 51.

6. Ibid, pp. 65-6.

7. Ibid, p. 51.

8. J.P. Byrne, *Encyclopedia of Pestilence, Pandemics and Plagues*, Santa Barbara: ABC-CLIO 2008, p. 519.

9. Boccaccio, *The Decameron*, trans. M. Rigg, London: David Campbell 1921, Vol I, pp. 5–11 (abridged).

10. Kelly, *The Great Mortality*, pp. 11-12.

11. Ibid, p. 22.

12. Author of *The Great Mortality*.

13. P.S. Sehdev, 'The Origin of Quarantine', *Clinical Infectious Diseases* 35 (9) PMID 12398064 (2002) pp. 1071-2.

14. Kelly, *The Great Mortality*, pp. 110-11.

15. Ibid, p. 152.

16. Ibid.

17. P. Daileader, *The Late Middle Ages* (audio course), Chantilly, Virginia:The Teaching Company 2007.

18. O.J. Benedictow, 'The Black Death: The Greatest Catastrophe Ever', *History Today,* Vol 55 (March 2005).

Chapter 4

1. P.M. Rogers, *Aspects of Western Civilisation*, Upper Saddle River: Pearson, 2000, p. 353-65.

2. *Eastern Mediterranean Health Journal*, Vol 23, issue 12, (2017).

3. R. Horrox, *The Black Death*, Manchester: Manchester University Press 1994, p. 15.

4. P. Ziegler, *The Black Death*, London: Penguin Books 1982, pp. 104-5.

5. Ibid, pp. 113-14.

6. Ibid, p. 19 (edited).

7. P. Papon, *De la Peste*, Paris : Lavillette & Cie 1799, Vol I, p. 115.

8. Ziegler, *The Black Death*, pp. 74-5.

9. Sulphur is still used to disinfect wine barrels before re-use.

10. Ziegler, *The Black Death*, pp. 53-5.

11. Ibid, pp. 57-8.

12. Ibid, p. 85, quoting G. Sticker, *Die Geschichte der Pest*, Töplemann: Giessen 1908, p. 68.

13. Quoted in Scott and Duncan, *Return of the Black Death*, p. 41.
14. Abridged excerpt from *The Annals of Ireland by Friar John Clyn*, ed. B. Williams, Dublin: Four Courts Press 2007.
15. Abridged extract from John of Fordoun, *Chronicle of the Scottish Nation,* ed. W.F. Skene, Edinburgh, Scottish Text Society 1872.
16. Kelly, *The Great Mortality*, p. 343-4.
17. Ziegler, *The Black Death*, p. 246.
18. Quoted in Scott and Duncan, *Return of the Black Death*, p. 90.
19. Quoted in Ibid, p. 92.
20. Quoted in Ibid.

Chapter 5

1. Article by B. Guarino in *Washington Post* 16 January 2018.
2. Ibid, *The Great Mortality*, p. 26.
3. Quoted in Scott and Duncan, *Return of the Black Death*, pp. 11, 13.
4. Ibid, p. 12.
5. Ibid, pp. 15, 16 (abridged).
6. Ibid, p. 19 (abridged).
7. Ibid, p. 21 (abridged).
8. Ibid, p. 25.
9. N. Cummins, M. Kelly and C. Ó Gráda, 'Living Standards and Plague in London 1560–1665', *English Historical Review* 69 (1), on which much of this section is based.
10. Scott and Duncan, *Return of the Black Death*, pp. 70-1 (quotation abridged).
11. Ibid, p. 78.
12. Ibid, p. 6 (original spelling).
13. Ibid, p. 7.
14. Ibid, pp. 82, 84.
15. C.J. Duncan and S. Scott, 'What Caused the Black Death?', *British Medical Journals /Postgraduate Medical Journal*, Vol 81 Issue 955 (2005).
16. D. Boyd, *Lionheart: The True Story of England's Crusader King*, Stroud: The History Press 2015, pp. 144-264.

17. First published in 1556.
18. Zinsser *Rats, Lice and History*, pp. 81-3.

Chapter 6

1. Article by J.S. Merrill in *Encyclopedia Brittanica on line.*
2. Also known as Barbara Villiers, the countess of Castlemaine and duchess of Cleveland in her own right.
3. All the quotations from the diary are to be found on line at https:// www.pepysdiary/diary. Many have been abridged here.
4. 'alone with her I tried to have my way and did so despite her resistance, but not to my complete satisfaction.'
5. King James I had ordered these to be built; also pest houses in Oxford, Newcastle and Windsor.
6. Scott and Duncan, *Return of the Black Death*, p. 37.
7. The quotations from John Evelyn's diary are taken from *The Diary of John Evelyn*, Vol II, a facsimile edition of the edition of 1901, published by Lector House, Delhi. Some have been abridged.
8. Byrne, *Encyclopedia of the Black Death*, pp. 208-10.
9. Ibid, pp. 217-18.
10. Ibid, p. 321.
11. Ibid.
12. Ibid.
13. Ibid, pp. 120-1.
14. C. Wright, *The Dark Traveller*, London: Lulu Press Inc., p. 54.
15. Byrne, *Encyclopedia of the Black Death*, p. 343-4.
16. Ibid.
17. A full wig, word derived from the French *perruque.*

Chapter 7

1. D. Defoe, *A Journal of the Plague Year*, ed. C. Wall, London: Penguin 2003, p. 267.
2. Ibid, p. 268.
3. Byrne, *Encyclopedia of the Black Death*, pp. 38-46.
4. Ibid, p. 75.
5. Ibid, p. 174.

6. Ibid, pp. 76-7.
7. A. Wear, *The Western Medical Tradition 800 BC to AD 1800*, Cambridge: Cambridge University Press, p. 233-6.
8. Byrne, *Encyclopedia of the Black Death*, p. 271-2.
9. Ibid, pp. 175-6.
10. Ibid.
11. Known as Marriotte's Law in France.
12. Byrne, *Encyclopedia of the Black Death*, pp. 334-5.
13. Wear, *The Western Medical Tradition*, pp. 233-6.
14. Byrne, *Encyclopedia of the Black Death*, pp. 333-4, 363.
15. Ibid, pp. 310-12.
16. Ibid, p. 339.
17. Ibid, pp. 310-12.

Chapter 8

1. G.D. Sussman's article in *Journal of World History*, Vol. 27 2016, p. 253.
2. According to a memorial in the church.
3. Article by D. McKenna in *BBC News* 5 November 2016.
4. Byrne, *Encyclopedia of the Black Death*, pp. 217-18.
5. M.D. Grmek and H.H. Mollaret, *Histoire de la Pensée Médicale en Occident*, Vol II, Paris: Seuil 1997, p. 376.
6. J-N Biraben, *Les Hommes et la Peste en France et dans les pays européens et méditerranéens*, Paris: La Haye 1975, p. 407.
7. Colbert's famous last words, after refusing a visit from Louis XVI on his deathbed, were, 'If I had done for God what I have done for that man, I should be saved ten times over.'
8. F. Lebrun, *Se soigner autrefois, médecins, saints et sorciers aux 17e et 18e siècles*, Paris: Messidor, pp. 161-4.

Chapter 9

1. Pepys' strange reference to a fainting woman may be his way of referring to what Bloodworth was reputed to have said when woken to see the fire in its early stages. It was, 'Pish. A woman could piss it out,' before going back to bed.

Chapter 10

1. Letter from Thomas Wade to Williamson, dated Whitby, 14 September.
2. Parliamentary Archives, HL/PO/PU/1/1666/18&19C2n14.
3. E.A. Wrigley and R.S. Schofield, *The Population History of England 1541–1871*, London: Hodder & Stoughton 1981.
4. Prince Rupert of the Rhine was a grandson of King James I and had been a Cavalier leader before being exiled. He returned to England at the Restoration.
5. Londoners and visitors interested in the plague pits can find comprehensive information on www.historic-uk.com/History Magazine/DestinationsUK/Londonplaguepits.

Chapter 11

1. Defoe, *A Journal of the Plague Year,* pp. 94-5.
2. Zinsser, *Rats, Lice and History*, pp. 159-60.
3. See D. Boyd, *The French Foreign Legion*, Hersham: Ian Allan Publishing 2010, pp. 102-12.
4. A *lazaretto*, named after the Biblical character Lazarus, revered as the patron saint of lepers, was a quarantine hospital at a port with facilities for fumigation of baggage and search of whole ships and their cargoes.

Chapter 12

1. See article by Rebecca Maki downloadable from www.antimicrobe. org/h04c.files/history/yersinia-pestis.asp.
2. McNeill, *Plagues and Peoples*, pp. 165-6.
3. Report by K.R Dean, F. Krauer and B.V. Schmid, downloadable from royalsocietypublishing.org/doi/10.1098/rsos.181695.
4. Report by G. Sharpe on BBC Scotland 31 August 2013.
5. http://emedicine.medscape.com/article/226871.
6. Wright, *The Long and Complicated Relationship between Humans and Yersinia Pestis.*

Chapter 13

1. Hippocrates *Epidemics* Vol I i, quoted by McNeill, *Plagues and Peoples*, p. 318.
2. Ibid.
3. D. Boyd, *April Queen: Eleanor of Aquitaine*, Stroud: The History Press 2011, pp. 114-15.
4. Boyd, *Lionheart*, pp. 196-8.
5. Boyd, *The French Foreign Legion*, pp. 173-4 and as an e-book.
6. D. Boyd, *The Other First World War*, Stroud: The History Press 2014, pp. 104-5, 115-16, 206-8, 210-13, 216-19, 223-4, 238.

Chapter 14

1. Scott and Duncan, *Return of the Black Death*, p. 283.
2. S. Milligan, *Scorflufus* poem. Downloadable from http//monologues, co.uk.
3. See *New England Journal of Medicine*, Issue 383 (8 October 2020), pp. 1479-1480; DOI: 10.1056/NEJM2029812 (abbreviated).
4. Article by Robert Wallgate published online 27 April 2004 (abridged).

Chapter 15

1. K. Alibek and S. Handelman, *Biohazard*, New York: Random House 2000, p. 112.
2. Wills, *Plagues*, pp. 21-2, 250.
3. Ibid, p. 253.
4. Ibid, pp. 31-3, 35.
5. Alibek and Handelman, *Biohazard*.
6. Scott and Duncan, *Return of the Black Death*, pp. 290-1.

Chapter 16

1. J. Lovelock, *The Ages of Gaia: A Biography of Our Living Earth*, New York: Bantam 1990, p. 22.
2. M. de Montaigne, *Essais*, Bordeaux 1580.

3. Full title: J. Lovelock, *The Revenge of Gaia: Why the Earth Is Fighting Back – and How We Can Still Save Humanity*, Santa Barbara: Allen Lane 2006.
4. It was a different age: they were paid $5,000 for appearing!
5. The name Gaia was suggested to Lovelock by his neighbour, the novelist William Golding.
6. Named after William Hyde Wollaston FRS (1766–1828).
7. Wills, *Plagues*, pp. 251, 291-3.

Appendix

1. Wills, *Plagues*, p. 239.
2. Ibid, p. 235.
3. Ibid, p. 218.
4. Ibid, p. 244.
5. Scott and Duncan, *Return of the Black Death*, p. 260.
6. C. Moorehead, *Gellhorn*, New York: Holt 2003, pp. 191-2.
7. Wills, *Plagues*, pp. 17-8.
8. Report in *La Voz de Galicia*, 30 June 2020.

Index